To
Lawrence

    I got you this book
    Since you seem to
    be dreaming of Sexual
happenings.

        love you

        Lisa xx
            x

UNDERSTANDING YOUR SEXUAL DREAMS

UNDERSTANDING YOUR SEXUAL DREAMS

by
Anna Treacher

SUNBURST BOOKS

This edition first published in 1995 by
Sunburst Books, Deacon House,
65 Old Church Street, London SW3 5BS

© 1995 Sunburst Books

ISBN 1-85778-182-1

Printed and bound in Finland

Contents

INTRODUCTION

By the time we die we will have spent more than a third of our lives sleeping. It may seem like a terrible waste of time when you consider how short life is, but sleep is necessary to allow the body to rejuvenate and repair cells. It is also important for the health of your mind.

When we sleep, we cannot prevent ourselves from dreaming, and indeed dreams perform an essential function in that they hold up a mirror to what is going on in our daily life. Whatever is preying on your mind will be reflected in your night-time slumbers.

Our dreams can show us how to lead fuller lives, to throw off the shackles of inhibition and fear and deal effectively with our problems. The realm of sleep can help to provide us with the answers we are seeking if we listen carefully.

However, bear in mind that very few dreams are literal depictions of our lives. The visions we see often leave us perplexed as they seem to be irrelevant. Yet think about the symbolism within your dreams and relate it to what is happening in your life and you will come closer to the message of the dream.

Sexual dreams — and the understanding of these lies at the heart of this book — often cause the most worry. People feel embarrassed by them, especially when they are doing things that they would – as they say – never dream of. Dreaming of being raped or of being the victim of incestuous abuse is a very frightening experience, yet the interpretation arrived at will not mean that the dreamer actually wants to experience these things.

Similarly, dreaming of stabbing someone to death does not mean that somewhere you have the urge to commit such a crime. More likely it means that you wish to destroy a part of yourself that makes you unhappy, and it is therefore a positive expression of your feelings.

This book aims to help you to open your eyes and mind to the new and often surprising vistas that the dream world can reveal to us. It will help you to unravel the message behind your dreams and give you an insight into that hidden yet very familiar half of your world. The result will be a better understanding of yourself and others.

Dreams use a language that is different from the one we use during our waking hours. Therefore it is important to be able to understand that language in order to make sense of the elaborate plots that are often woven into the fabric of our dreams.

Sexual Dreams does the groundwork for you by explaining in Chapter 1 what a dream is. It goes on to show the difference between fantasy and dreams, and looks at what happens during dreams and at why we dream in the first place.

Dream analysis is the subject of Chapter 2, which explains how to apply certain rules of interpretation to your own dreams. Analysing a dream is quite straightforward once you know what to look for. This chapter will take you step by step into your own dreamland so that you can become your own dream counsellor.

Chapter 3 is an A-Z directory of sexual dreams. After a brief introduction to the dreamer, her or his dream is described and an analysis of its meaning is given. In this way many different types of dreams are examined, as well as a wide range of personalities.

Dreams, whether they are sexual or otherwise, can be

grouped into specific recognised types. Problem-solving dreams, to take just one example, are among the most common of dreams. We use them to help us to iron out the kinks in our lives. They deal with issues that cause us conflict, and in the case of sexual dreams they can give us the answer to questions like 'Should I allow this relationship get more intimate?' The main types of dreams and their functions are looked at in detail in Chapter 4.

Even though every dream is unique to an individual, there are themes that crop up over and over again, and these are the subject of Chapter 5. The details within such a dream differ from person to person, but the main theme remains the same. A perfect and common example is falling. It can manifest itself in a dream as a person falling down stairs, from a building or out of a plane. A dream of this kind is telling the person that he or she is losing control of a worrying situation.

Every dream is littered with symbols which are important in deciphering the message of the dream. There are thousands of them — far too many to deal with in a book like this. For this reason, in Chapter 6 I have chosen those which are most common or have a particular relevance to sexual dreams.

Sexual dreams take many different guises. They can be gentle and serene, with just a subtle hint of virginal flesh on display; soft and romantic, with a discreetly stolen kiss the only sexual contact; or they can be raunchy, with scenes of rampant sex and orgies. Unfortunately they can also be frightening.

See if you can relate to any of the wide range of sexual dreams analysed in the A-Z directory. Some types of sexual dream crop up repeatedly and these are described here, among the many hundreds of other scenarios.

If you'd like to have your own sexual dreams and find it difficult to initiate them, then Chapter 7 can help. Here you will find out how to curb your inhibitions in order to create the perfect mood in which to drift off into a marvellous sexual dream.

Just as what you dream at night can help you to overcome your problems during the day, so sexual dreams can help you to pinpoint areas in your love-life which need working on. And although you probably already know – or at least suspect – they may be able to confirm that you are having problems within a relationship, and perhaps provide the catalyst to break the damaging bonds of a dead-end romance.

Sexual Dreams is not only great entertainment — I hope that it will also help you to make the most of your waking hours, and even change your destiny.

CHAPTER ONE

WHAT IS A DREAM?

We all, without exception, dream. People who say that they don't, probably never remember their dreams. Men are particularly unwilling to own up to dreaming, but the fact is that we can dream up to five times a night. Although we may not remember our dreams they are an important part of our lives, for without them our mental and physical health would be at risk.

Dreams usually occur during REM sleep. REM stands for Rapid Eye Movement. Scientists carrying out sleep experiments discovered that when rapid eye movement occurred, more often than not the subject was dreaming.

Rapid eye movement comes about when the dreamer 'watches' the activities that are happening during the dream, almost as though he or she were awake during the day. REM periods happen four or five times a night and start about an hour and a half after we first go to sleep. Each lasts between 10 and 45 minutes.

Using electronic monitoring equipment, scientists measuring the brain's impulses found that these impulses fluctuated. In waking hours they were of a low frequency, while in sleep they were high. 'Let me sleep on it' is not just an empty cliché. Research has shown that volunteers subjected to sleep deprivation find that their ability to cope with the trials and tribulations of everyday life is diminished to some degree, depending on the individual.

We become nervous and edgy when we experience sleep deprivation, and few people can tolerate more than three days and nights of being prevented from entering the dreaming state.

During sleep those images that make up a dream cause the body to react as though it were experiencing for real the event being dreamed about. Researchers have found that physical reactions include a raised heart rate, fluctuating blood pressure, increased blood flow and, in the cases of nightmares, the release into the body of adrenalin — the 'fight or flight' reaction — when faced with danger.

Even our muscles react, but fortunately only the minor ones that control our fingers and toes tend to twitch. Messages to the brain which would normally cause movement are inhibited by neurons in the stem of the brain.

However, only very rarely do we act out what is in our dreams. There have been a number of examples of so-called 'night terrors' where dreamers acted out their dreams with tragic consequences. In one case a man killed his wife while dreaming he was a samurai warrior.

There are also other more intimate parts of our bodies that react to dreams. Research has shown that during sexually arousing dreams a man will get an erection and a woman's vagina will become engorged.

Our imagination is central to our ability to dream. How often have we used it to create a pleasant daydream, or, just before we drop off to sleep, to recall a happy event? We use our imaginations to place ourselves at the scene of many things, imagining what it would be like to collect the degree we are working for, to be with someone we lust after. We even place ourselves for a while in the roles of actor and actresses in films we have seen.

We all fantasise at some stage in our lives. The difference between dreams and fantasies is that our dreams are spontaneous and not consciously controlled, whereas our fantasies are.

And yet it is possible to influence the content of our

dreams before we go to sleep by creating the right atmosphere and frame of mind. But as those who remember their dreams will testify, they do not follow a steady path. Instead the images jump around so that in one scene we can be enjoying a cup of tea at our kitchen table and in the next running down corridors in a strange building trying to get away from something horrendous that is pursuing us.

Anything can trigger a dream or nightmare. A romantic film, a magazine article on a famous pop group, an argument, a touch from a partner or pet, sounds or smells outside our sleeping world. But, just as often, it needs none of these outside stimuli to make us dream. Instead, the impulses come from within.

While we experience the dream it seems very real to us, but on waking and remembering it, we know that it was not daytime reality. 'It was only a dream,' we say, as though we had just been watching a video hired for the night. Expert opinion is divided when it come to deciding what a dream is and if indeed it really exists. Do we really touch a spiritual or psychic side of ourselves or are dreams merely the brain's way of 'downloading' information, of having a good clear-out, before the following day?

The universal experience of dreaming has been a source of interest for many centuries, and in a variety of cultures, but it was not until the late 1800s that dreams were studied in earnest in the Western world. Even then, psychologists differed greatly in their interpretation of the visions that sleep brings us. There were several schools of thought. One of these believed that we dream in symbols, everyday objects representing emotions, while another held that dreams are a form of escapism — rather like a cinema of the mind. Yet another said that dreaming was just a method of emptying the brain of undigested thoughts that were of no use to us.

The early part of the present century saw a plethora of papers by noted psychologists claiming to offer the definitive explanation of our dreams. Sigmund Freud and Carl Jung were the most renowned figures in this field. Their ideas about dreams are in complete opposition.

To put complex beliefs in simple terms, Freud held that dreams are a form of wish-fulfilment — a way of achieving a wish during our sleeping hours that we fail to achieve while awake because of our own repression. Everything in dreams has an alternative, coded meaning, and in order to understand a dream you must unlock this code through understanding the symbols it uses. Most of Freud's symbols related to sex because he believed dreams had their roots in sexual frustration. To analyse the dreams of his patients, he used 'free association', in which they spoke about the thoughts that these dreams evoked.

By contrast, Jung felt that dreams did not necessarily mean anything. He did not advocate free association and was of the opinion that whatever appeared in a dream was there not as a symbol but because it was merely an object in the dream. Unlike Freud, he felt that the overall content of a dream was more important than any one specific thing. Again by way of contrast, while Freud maintained that dreams hid the dreamer's secrets, Jung believed that they revealed them.

In our dreams any pretence is stripped away. Think back to some of the ludicrous situations in which you have found yourself in dreams — situations you would definitely avoid given the chance. For example, during waking hours you would never dream of appearing naked in front of work colleagues, yet in a dream it is entirely possible.

Dreams are valuable precisely because they show this

other side of ourselves. By thoroughly and honestly analysing their contents we can discover their true meaning. Dreams are a normal part of our life and whether we want to look into them or not, they will always be there. However, if we choose to do so, by treating them as part of a process of creative, lateral thinking we can help ourselves to understand everyday problems. In short, they help us to view our problems from a different angle and often provide us with a solution.

CHAPTER TWO

ANALYSING DREAMS

A dream does not unfold in an ordered, logical fashion. It cuts out things like walking from one part of a house to another or transposes you from sitting on a park bench to flying overhead in a hot-air balloon. And you will not be able to remember walking upstairs or getting into the balloon. As in Star Trek, you are 'beamed up' from one place or time to another. This is one of the main ways in which dreams differ from reality. Understanding this fact should help you avoid adopting too literal an approach to the interpretation of what occurs in your dreams.

A dream can be broken down into three key components. First, it places you in a time where your problem originated and you will recognise things that are synonymous with that era. Second, it shows you how your problem is surfacing in your life now. Finally, it presents you with an answer to the problem that you are experiencing. So, when you come to interpret your dream, look for those three key elements before moving on to deal with the next main component: dream symbols.

These symbols are important in that they pinpoint the message of a dream. In order to analyse a dream it is a good idea to familiarise yourself with the dream symbols. There are many thousands of these and in Chapter 3 I have given an alphabetical section listing some of the most common ones so that you can begin deciphering your own dreams.

When you begin to analyse your dreams it is important to bear in mind that every dream is self-specific. A dream is made up of many different facets, all of which reflect the dreamer's personality and life experience. It is possible for two people to have dreams with the same key symbols in them, but the interpretation of the two dreams will necessarily be different because they are not the same person.

Therefore the message that a dream holds is specifically for you. Dreams are in effect private messages which only you, the dreamer, will truly understand as they are created by your unconscious mind.

Even so, at first it will be difficult to interpret the dream and you will wonder what relevance certain symbols have for you. It will seem like a foreign language, but you will learn. Don't give up because once you have cracked the code then you will benefit from the solution. It may seem unnecessary to say this, but once you have the solution, act on it.

Those of us who tend to remember our dreams do so in two ways – either in scraps where key words log in our mind, or in considerable detail. However, it is highly unlikely that you will remember every single element of the dream unless you wake up in the middle of it or just as it finishes. This makes it all the more important, in order to get the maximum practical benefit out of your dream, not to ignore any clue it offers.

The first step towards analysing a dream is to recall and record it, and I will show you how to do this in a few simple steps. Create a dream manual — this can be any book of plain paper which is set aside for dreams only. Before you go to sleep, jot down a few detail about events that day. Note how you felt. There is no need to go into great detail. These notes are necessary for helping to interpret your dreams later.

Now decide how you want to record your dream. You

can either use a tape recorder or a pen and paper. In choosing a method, bear in mind how you usually feel first thing in the morning. Writing down the details may seem like too much hard work at first light.

If you decide to use a tape recorder, speak into it as though you were recounting the dream to someone else. It doesn't matter if it comes out a little jumbled; just say whatever comes into your mind at the time. The analysis will help to sort it out later.

If you sleep with someone, then using a small torch will ensure that your partner is not unduly disturbed by your scribbling.

Are you determined to remember your dream? One way of ensuring that you do is to concentrate hard on it just before you go to sleep. Sit on the side of the bed and relax for a while before focusing your mind on your goal and then say firmly, 'Tonight I will sleep. I will dream. I will remember it in the morning.'

Then make sure your pen and paper or tape recorder are close at hand and lie down and go to sleep.

As I explained earlier, it is quite possible for someone to have up to five dreams a night. Initially you may wake up after more than one dream. While it might seem irksome to have to record your dream at 3.30 a.m., nevertheless steel yourself and do it. Once you have become more practised at it, you will know instinctively know which dreams really have a message for you.

When it comes to recalling the dream, it is a good idea not to jump up immediately to record the details. Just lie there for a minute or two and allow the memory of the dream to wash over you. Then write or record everything that comes to mind. It can be anything from specific detail, through to taste, colour or smell. Recall how you felt or feel — fear, disgust, pleasure, for example — the mood of the dream. If possible, note the time when you woke as well.

Keep your dreams in your dream manual so that you can refer to them and gradually build up an overall picture which will reveal whether there is a pattern to your dream life. Transfer any taped dreams into the manual when you are fully awake.

Now look at your dream and note the key symbols, which may be anything from objects to animals to colours, emotions, actions, smells or noises. Ring them with a different-coloured pen so that they stand out. Now look up the symbols in Chapter 6. You will find that there will be a series of different options for each heading. Note them down and eventually you will have an alternative picture of your dream. It is here that its message lies.

Remember that the message is specific to you, so do not rely absolutely on what the symbols mean. By looking back on the notes you made of what happened the day before the dream, and incorporating this in the analysis, you will be able to interpret the message more accurately.

The main difficulty with dream analysis is deciding which dream symbol is relevant to you. However, there are a few important points to keep in mind and some basic symbols that occur all the time and have direct relevance to the dreamer's personality and experiences.

For example, dreaming of a child may represent the juvenile part of you, while dreaming of an older person may represent the part that is ageing or growing wiser. Other people frequent our dreams, but focus on what qualities they have and which ones are dominant because, more often than not, the people in your dream represent aspects of yourself.

Dreaming of being male or female is directly related to your own male and female sides. Animals refer to characteristics associated with them. For example, the presence of a duck or ducks, calling to mind the saying 'water off a duck's back', means that nothing really bothers you.

Buildings such as houses represent yourself, each room standing for different emotions and aspects of your personality. The cellar or basement is connected to your sexuality; the ground floor, your physical being; and the upper rooms or attic, your spirituality.

If these symbols appear in you dream, don't take them on face value, but examine how they affect you or represent you.

Finally, to make the important procedure of dream-recording as effective as possible, use the following simple checklist. The better you recall you dreams, the better equipped you will be to analyse them.

1. In your dream manual, jot down some details from the previous day.

2. Put a notebook and pen or tape recorder beside your bed.

3. Sit on the side of your bed and tell yourself you will remember your dreams.

4. Record any dreams as soon as you wake up.

5. Record your feelings during the dream and after.

6. Note the key symbols.

7. Refer to Chapter 6 to find the general meanings of dream symbols.

8. Apply these meanings to your current situation or problem.

At the end of this book there are a number of pages available for you to use for your dream notes.

CHAPTER THREE

A-Z OF SEXUAL DREAMS

Own up those of you who have had sexual dreams but have been too shy, embarrassed or ashamed to confess to them. Bringing up the very subject of sex is bound to make some of your friends or colleagues feel uncomfortable. But to tell them that you had a sexy, maybe even perverted dream last night — well, it's just not what they were expecting to hear, is it?

Although we may not have as many sexual dreams as other types of dreams, they are an important part of our dream world and hence reflect on our everyday life. However, it doesn't mean you are a pervert just because you dream of having sex with your father or mother; nor does it necessarily mean you have homosexual leanings if you dream of a raunchy encounter with someone of your own sex.

Sexual dreams often have nothing to do with sex but are the mind's way of getting us to address other unrelated problems in our life. Just as importantly, they can also be a way of letting you know that all is well. Symbolism plays a big part in these dreams as in any other kind of dream, but don't automatically assume that if you dream of what is universally seen as a phallic symbol, that the dream must be about sex. In some dreams the penis represents creativity.

When analysing a sexual dream – as with any kind of dream – remember that the message it contains is for you and reflects the way you feel and how you deal with situations in your life. Sexual dreams evoke powerful feelings in the dreamer — not just in a sexual way, but in the way she or he feels about what is actually happening in the dream. When recalling the dream, pay particular attention to these emotions and write them down.

The remainder of this chapter consists of a wide-ranging collection of sexual dreams and their analysis. Read about them carefully and see how the technique of dream analysis is put to work in each case. Do any of these dreams ring a bell with you? Try to analyse them for yourself before reading the conclusion. This will help to prepare for the challenge of examining your own dreams.

ADAM AND EVE

Louise is a 17-year-old student. She has been seeing Karl for six months and she's crazy about him. An A- level student, she has plans to go to university.

Karl is very laid-back and – while not exactly a rebel – he is very creative and hopes to go to art college. He is constantly telling Louise how much he loves her. She feels the same way, although when it comes to sex they have very different ideas.

Brought up by strict parents, Louise has an ingrained belief that she should wait until she gets married before she has sex. Karl, on the other hand, thinks that they should become more intimate. Louise had a dream not long after a row with him about the subject.

THE DREAM

It was like something out of paradise. I was standing in a pool of crystal-clear water; the sun was beating down and I felt good as I submerged myself. My hair was long and golden and as I rose from the pool I was naked.

I climbed on to the bank and lay on the green grass, warming myself like a cat drinking in the heady, sweet smells of exotic flowers. As I lay there I saw a young, well-built man ease himself into the pool. He didn't know I was there, and as I watched he scooped up the water in his hands and poured it over his face. It ran in rivulets down his honed body, over his navel and manhood, and continued down his taut legs. I was fascinated by him and could feel desire stirring deep inside me.

He lay back in the pool and as I watched I knew I had

to touch and taste him. Later when he climbed out of the water I followed him through the lush green jungle, but after a few steps he used to disappear into thin air.

This happened for what seemed like days in a row — in my dream the same scene was played over and over again. I'd lie on the bank watching him. Once or twice he turned around and it seemed as though he was listening as if he knew I was watching him.

Then one day as I followed him through the jungle and this time he didn't disappear, but climbed a tree and, reaching out his arms, tried to grab the fruit that was growing on it. It fell to the ground and he followed after, crashing his head on a rock as he fell. I held my breath, waiting for him to move, but he didn't.

I was nervous, but I crept up to his still body and prodded it, but there was no movement. I couldn't work out if he was breathing or not, so I put my head on his chest. It was hairless and still warm.

The object of his desire lay beside him — an apple — but it was bruised and gashed. As I reached across his body to pick it up he suddenly awoke, and when I looked at his eyes they were those of a snake and as he spoke a serpent-type tongue flickered in and out of his mouth. I was absolutely shocked and I woke with a start from my dream.

ANALYSIS

The Adam and Eve connotation is very obvious, except that in Louise's dream she has not gone the whole way. Although she feels deep emotion for Karl, she is scared to go one step further and commit her body to him.

The presence of the jungle, with its beautiful, exotic sounds and smells, shows that she is on the threshold of discovery. The apple has long had special connotations, most notably of lust. In Louise's dream, it is never consumed, and therefore her sexual needs remain unfulfilled.

She is ambitious and sees Karl as someone who, although he is great to be with, could lead her astray, so that she neglected her ambitions. She should cool the relationship with him as she clearly isn't ready to give all of herself yet.

ADULTERY

A personal assistant to a foreign editor, Tina moved to London last year with her boyfriend, who is a student. Her boyfriend took a year off from his studies to come to London, but in two months' time he has to return to Germany to finish his degree course. Tina is staying in England.

The couple are convinced that their relationship will survive the separation and plan to spend as much time as possible together in the months leading up to his departure. However, lately they have started to bicker about little things — something they never used to do. Tina cannot understand why at a time like this they should be behaving in this way. She finds it difficult to be close to her boyfriend sexually, even though she admits that she loves him deeply.

Her dream shows her involved with someone else, although this is something she has never done in the five years they have been together.

THE DREAM

I am at the airport and it is busy with people rushing to catch their planes. My boyfriend and I are standing with our arms wrapped around each other and I am crying. He tells me not to cry and that in a few months' time we will see each other again. Almost hysterically, I say, 'That's not good enough.'

A pained look crosses his face and he says, 'You will wait for me,' to which I reply, 'Of course I will.' As he walks down the ramp to join the rest of the passengers I stand there, tears pouring down my face.

In the next scene I am lying on a sofa half naked, kissing a man. The lights are low and I am particularly wild with him, undoing his clothes and urging him to take them off until we are both naked. All this time we are kissing. He says, 'Let's go to the bedroom,' and it's then that I look at him and as I do so, I realise it is not my boyfriend. I start sobbing and grab my clothes to my chest, desperately trying to put them on.

When I wake up, my boyfriend is shaking me gently, saying, 'It's all right.' I had been crying in my sleep. That dream really disturbed me but I didn't tell him about it.

ANALYSIS

Although Tina is not married, she is in a committed relationship. Adultery in a dream indicates a number of things, quite often guilt. Tina is perhaps feeling guilty that she is not going back to Germany with her boyfriend. It also indicates a problem of a sexual nature in a relationship — in their case it is probably only a temporary difficulty caused by the strain of her boyfriend's leaving.

The airport scene may well be just a reflection of what is going to happen in reality. However, airports can symbolise great change, and Tina may be about to change direction in her life.

ANAL SEX

Fiona has been married for 10 years. Now 35, she is being constantly reminded by family and friends alike that her biological clock is ticking away. Lately, even her husband, Tony, has begun to talk about having children. She finds the pressure is getting to her and feels quite angry that people have set themselves up as judge of what she should do with her life.

Added to all this pressure is Fiona's recent promotion to the position of advertising director. This responsibility is something that she has worked hard for and she is justifiably proud of her achievement. She knows that pregnancy at this stage of her career would be fatal and she has developed a phobia about contraception, often faking a headache so that she does not have to make love with her husband.

THE DREAM
I have had a dream about anal sex. It's the second time it has been the subject of my dreams. I have never tried it for real, although that doesn't mean to say I don't have a varied and fulfilling sex life — it's just that it has never really appealed to me.

I am on holiday with Tony at what looks like a Caribbean resort. It is evening time and we have just finished our dinner. As we walk along the shoreline of the beach we are holding hands and kissing every now and then. Sitting on the sand, we listen to the sound of the waves, our arms around each other.

As we sit there he puts his hand under my chin and

starts to kiss me passionately, his tongue probing my mouth. I respond and his fingers work their way inside my blouse, teasing my erect nipples. Without a word and still embracing each other urgently, we go back to our hotel room, where within seconds our naked bodies are writhing under a shower of deliciously warm water.

As we become more and more aroused, he sits in the bath and beckons me to come and sit on him, but when I do I find I have no vagina for him to enter and instead we have anal sex. Neither of us seems to be particularly disturbed by this.

It is strange that I should have a dream like this. Does it mean that I want a more adventurous love-life?

ANALYSIS

A dream that has the anus as its main focal point indicates rebellion in the dreamer. Looking back on what Fiona has said is preying on her mind. It could be that she is acting out her feelings about all the pressure she is under to have a baby. It is her way of asserting herself once and for all.

The lack of a vagina could well indicate her reluctance to get pregnant, it being the only route to pregnancy. On a more positive note, the presence of water in the form of the ocean indicates her sexual desire for her husband and is a positive symbol.

APHRODISIACS

Nick is a 44-year-old quantity surveyor. Twice divorced, he has now been without a partner for the past year. It isn't for lack of effort on his part — he just never seems to click with any of the women he meets.

Three months ago Nick joined a dating agency and has already replied to five of the women who contacted him. But each time he met up with them nothing happened, and the last time in particular was an absolute disaster, shattering his already fragile ego.

'I had seen this woman three times and on the third time, after a heavy necking session at my place, she reached down and placed her hand inside my trousers, to be met with a lukewarm reception. She was obviously very miffed and asked me if I found her attractive. I told her I did, but she replied, "Well, why doesn't that work then?" Needless to say that was the last time I saw her.'

About a week later Nick had the following dream.

THE DREAM

Suddenly I was in the middle of what seemed to be a tribal or voodoo ceremony. It was pitch black and the air was filled with the aromatic smell of burning wood. Around me, fearsome painted faces pushed close to mine as they mumbled something to me in a funny language.

I felt afraid but somehow exhilarated and I let two tribesmen with ramrod-straight backs lead me into a shanty-town type of house. A wizened old man sat on a low stool. He spoke to me in English and told me he could give me my heart's desire.

As he said that, he nodded towards a doorway and told me to look through it. As I did I saw a powerfully built man straddled by a woman with a curvy body grinding against him until she was exhausted and another woman had to take her place. This procession of women went on and on and the man showed no signs of flagging.

A hand on my shoulder turned me around and the witch doctor smiled a broken-toothed smile at me and said, 'You want, yes?'

He led me, nodding to a table laid out with a variety of potions in tiny bowls. The only thing I recognised were oysters — the rest were powders and creams. After saying some mumbo-jumbo over them, he said, 'Eat.'

I did what he said, grabbing everything and cramming into my mouth, even though it tasted horrible. After gorging myself, I smiled smugly and walked out of the hut door into bright lights and the sound of laughing voices.

Standing there were what seemed like all the women in my life, laughing at me and pointing to my penis. As I slowly looked down, I saw it had shrunk to nothing. I could barely see it.

I woke up shouting, 'No-o-o-o.'

ANALYSIS

Nick's dream reflects his performance anxieties and his need for a quick fix.

It may be that a poor sex life was in part to blame for the breakdown of his marriage. His eagerness to accept the array of aphrodisiacs presented to him may indicate his refusal to acknowledge that his problems in holding down a relationship are probably more deep-rooted than anything any potion can solve.

His lack of self-esteem is directly connected to the withering process his penis went through. He might be wise to not try so hard to find a mate but instead spend time seeking other interests. When the right love comes along, everything will fall into place.

BESTIALITY

Jason is a 22-year-old virgin. As a teenager he was shy and self-conscious, so never had much luck with girlfriends. Instead he threw himself into his studies and eventually found his way into accountancy.

'I suppose I'm exactly what people expect of accountants,' he says apologetically. His face still bears the faint scars of teenage acne and his large blue eyes look out from behind heavy-framed glasses.

He doesn't smile easily and his constant hitching of his glasses up his nose gives away his nervousness in the company of women. Although he is no extrovert, once he starts talking about something that interests him he becomes animated.

At the moment he is not dating, but he harbours a secret crush for his immediate boss. Sylvia is 10 years older than him and a very confident woman; indeed, she could even be described as having a dominant personality.

'I dream a lot,' Jason reveals. 'Maybe it's because I don't sleep very well. Recently I have started to dream about work, nothing unusual, just about everyday, boring stuff. But a few weeks back I had a weird dream involving Sylvia. When I woke up I felt like a pervert.'

THE DREAM
I was in the office involved in a particularly tedious bit of calculation when Sylvia came over to my desk and slammed a folder down. I was so engrossed that I jumped and the total of the figures I had been calculating just disappeared out of my mind.

35

I don't mind telling you I was livid, but I didn't say anything, as usual. She sat on the corner of my desk, and in
the process knocked the pot of pens onto the floor. As I
scrabbled to the floor to get them, she addressed me. I
looked up and as I did I could see the tops of her stockings, deep and lacy, and a hint of flesh.

I started to stutter and one of the guys in the office saw
what was going on. He was in his mid-twenties and drove
a Porsche. He was the complete opposite to the stereo-
type of an accountant — a real high-flyer, in fact. He
swaggered over to my desk and putting his hand on
Sylvia's elbow, said 'Sylvia, dear, I think you've got an
admirer for life. You are the woman of Jason's dreams.'

Sylvia stood up, straightened her tight black skirt over
her thighs and, walking into her office to answer her
phone, said over her shoulder, 'Well, he can dream on.'

Everybody in the office laughed and I could feel myself
shrinking inside.

Then the dream shifted and we were at the office
party. I had had a lot to drink and became very chatty. 'I
always thought you were such a mouse,' said Amanda, the
section's secretary.

'I'm a lion,' I answered. But as I looked at her I saw her
eyes widen and she backed off, mumbling something
about the ladies' room.

I followed her down the hall, passing our office on the
way. From inside I could hear moans. The door was slightly ajar, so I peered in. When my eyes became accustomed
to the dim light I was absolutely shocked. There was
Sylvia, dressed in just a basque and stockings, locked in a
passionate embrace with what looked like a half man, half
ram. It had its back to me.

She was having sex with it across my desk and she

looked as if she was really enjoying herself. As she ran her red-painted nails across the arching back of the man-beast, she tilted her head back and I heard her sigh, 'Oh, Jase, you are so good.'

But what rooted me to the spot even more was when the creature turned around and I was looking at my own grinning face.

At work the day after I had that dream, I couldn't even look at Sylvia and I was so embarrassed that I feigned sickness to get off early.

ANALYSIS

Jason's shyness is crippling him in every aspect of his life. The presence of an animal in a dream is a potent form of symbolism. The ram is symbolic of virility, and the Zodiac sign Aries is represented by this creature. Arians are renowned for their assertiveness. Jason craves both to be sexually attractive and to get his own way in his work, hence the lovemaking taking place over his desk.

BONDAGE

Michelle is a 32-year-old housewife with two young children under the age of five. She is married to Neil, who works long hours in the City. She has a beautiful home in a private housing estate in Kent, but the mortgage is high.

She originally worked as a fashion PR, but gave that up to look after the children. With only a year between them, soon her son will be joining his older sister at primary school. Michelle feels she is at a crossroads in her life and is not sure what to do next.

Her sex life is stable — if you call sex twice a month stable. Neil is often too tired to make love when he comes home and even when they do manage to get it together, it leaves her feeling dissatisfied.

'Rather than thinking of England, I build fantasies in my head,' she admits. Often these fantasies spill into her dreams. 'There is one I always seem to be having — it involves bondage, which is strange because I've never tried it.'

THE DREAM

I'm in a bedroom, only it's not mine. The air is warm and the only source of light is from a cluster of burning white candles, giving the room a lovely cosy glow.

There is a bed in the centre of the room; it's a brass bed and the candlelight is reflected in it. There is nothing else in the room apart from the bed.

As I walk in a man gets up from it and walks towards me His face isn't clear to me, but I'm not frightened. He is tall – taller than me – and very masculine, with a tanned, well-developed body.

He reaches out to rip off the floaty black negligée I am wearing. Then, grabbing me by the hand, he pulls me to the bed and pushes me on to it. It is covered in a satiny fabric which is cool to the touch at first. As I lie there he straddles my stomach. He is naked and has an erection.

Leaning across me, he ties one hand, then the next to the bed posts, then he turns his body around, and leaning towards the end of the bed, he pulls my legs apart and ties each to a post.

I feel a sense of disappointment. The thought that he is just going to use me crosses my mind. Instead he kisses me on the neck and works his way down my body to plant kisses all over every part, including my feet.

Then after kissing and sucking my nipples, he runs his tongue down to my clitoris and stays there until he brings me to a climax.

When I come I feel all the tension leave my body and immediately fall asleep, only to be woken by him doing the same thing again until I come. I feel my bonds becoming loose and I run my fingers through his hair, keeping him at my clitoris as he satisfies me over and over again.

Eventually I let him go and he covers me with a satin sheet as I fall into a deep sleep.

When I woke in the morning after that dream I felt relaxed and whenever I thought about it during the day, I could feel myself getting turned on.

ANALYSIS

Michelle needs spoiling. She is disillusioned with her husband's approach to sex, which he treats it as a chore that has to be performed.

The ropes represent the way she feels about life at the moment: tied down and helpless. She is sexually restricted in her everyday life, but in her dreams she eventually takes control by being selfish about her own needs. It's something that she would never do in reality.

But now that the kids are away at school, she will have more time on her hands, and perhaps she ought to look at ways of encouraging her husband to take a more active role in lovemaking.

BREASTS

Alan has just moved back home to his parents' home after the break-up of his three-year-old marriage. His wife, Elaine, accused him of being immature during their often turbulent relationship. His response to any arguments has always been to walk out of the house, sometimes for hours, often for days, staying at his mother's home.

Recently Alan had a dream.

THE DREAM

I was in a pub with about five of my friends. We were playing a game of pool in the corner. It was a very noisy place, full of smoke with the jukebox blaring all the time.

It seemed like a normal evening. The crowd was mainly young, not trendy — just your average crowd. We were all drinking beer, and by about nine o'clock were pleasantly merry. A few girls had started to dance among themselves; they were getting drunk as well. It was somebody's birthday and it looked as if it was a girls' night out. There were some real lookers in the group — all dolled up.

My mate Martin gave me a nudge and shouted above the din, 'I reckon they're on the pull — we could get lucky here.'

He smiled over at them and I saw two smile back. All of a suddenly the song 'Patricia the Stripper' came on and a huge shout went up all over the pub.

A blonde-haired girl had taken off her top and was swinging it over her head, and then another in her group followed suit before they helped each other to take their bras off.

I stood there with my eyes glued to their breasts. I remember thinking they were beautiful. One by one all of the girls in the group started to undress, but only as far as the waist.

I walked to the bar to get a refill and even the barmaids were standing there bare-chested. 'Yeah, love, what can I get you?' one of them said, completely unabashed.

I was gobsmacked. I turned around to tell the lads, but when I did they were no longer there. All I could see was a sea of boobs.

I was the only man in the whole pub. The women moved towards me, smiling and one of them took my hand and held it to her breast, then another followed until I was completely surrounded by topless women pushing their bodies against me.

I was like a kid in a sweet shop. I had never seen so many different shapes and sizes and they were so soft to touch. They started to spin me around and around until their pink flesh was just a blur.

As I slowed down and began to refocus, all of the girls had grown older, much older — they seemed to be in their fifties and sixties and their boobs had begun to sag.

Then I suddenly woke up to the sound of my radio alarm. I had to laugh when I heard what song was playing. That's right, 'Patricia the Stripper'.

ANALYSIS

Alan's wife, Elaine, may have hit a nerve when she branded him immature. The presence of breasts in a man's dream more often than not simply indicates a sexual dream. However, in Alan's case it is significant that he should have this dream at the time that he has returned to the 'bosom' of his mother, leaving behind a disastrous marriage. He's a real mummy's boy.

Alan should ask himself whether he is mature enough to sustain an adult relationship, with all the responsibility that it entails. In his case the sea of breasts could well mean that he saw his wife as someone who fulfilled his need for a mother figure, someone to give him the maternal affection and care he craved.

He should beware, because a mother figure can easily become a smother figure.

CARESSING

Rebecca is a very talented writer who has always been unlucky in love. Self-obsessed, she is always trying to think of ways to change her life for the better, but she swings like a pendulum in her attempts. Her latest efforts have seen her give up cigarettes and alcohol and so far she has managed to do without both for more than four months.

She has also embarked on a healthy diet in a effort to shed the pounds she has gained from trying to comfort a broken heart by overeating.

THE DREAM
I am lying on a huge bed; it's so big that I cannot see over the sides. Everything is pink and fluffy and I'm looking gorgeous and glamorous. My recent ex-boyfriend is lying beside me smiling and looking deep into my eyes. He tells me that I am beautiful and reaches to touch my arm.

I feel so loved as he runs his masculine hands over my body and kisses the top of my head tenderly. He keeps whispering, saying things like, 'You are the most beautiful woman in the world,' and like a cat that is being stroked I am almost purring with pleasure. He caresses my bare arms and tells me that I have wonderful soft skin. That is all that the dream is about — just me being caressed.

ANALYSIS
Rebecca's dream reflects what she would really want in her daily life: to be loved and told that she is perfect. To

be caressed is to be loved and revered. She is full of self-doubt about herself and she needs to learn to accept herself and love herself before anyone else can.

CORPORAL PUNISHMENT

Lynn is a 24-year-old scientific research assistant in a large laboratory. Her father is a brilliant scientist and encouraged his only child to develop an interest in the field. She remembers that when she was a youngster he used to sit her on his knee and read from scientific journals, encouraging her to ask questions.

'To be perfectly honest, I would have preferred to have played with my dolls and cook a pretend dinner for them. But I knew that it made him happy, particularly when I'd quickly grasp what it was he was trying to explain.'

Although Lynn admits she is nowhere near as talented as her father, she does have an aptitude for the work. However, she has to try very hard and often feels as though the whole thing is a chore. Lately she has been toying with the idea of changing career, but she is not sure what to do.

THE DREAM

I am in a classroom. The chairs are tiny, as are the desks, and I am standing in a corner facing the wall a few feet away from the blackboard. I don't know why I am there but I've obviously been naughty. The teacher is a man and he is wearing a traditional black cloak over his clothes.

Every now and then I sneak a look over my shoulder and a row of tiny faces are intently watching him as he writes in white chalk on the board. The chalk squeaks in an irritating manner, sometimes making rude noises, which sends up a titter in the class.

He's a very grumpy teacher and keeps telling everyone

to keep quiet, sit straight, pay attention. My legs are aching and it seems like I have been there for eternity when the school bell goes. The shrillness of the sound makes me jump. I turn to go back to my desk to collect my school bag, but the teacher shouts, 'Stay and face the wall!'

I am not a child in my dream; I am an adult. Still facing the wall, I hear the rest of the class scraping their chairs along the black and white tiled floor and then the sound of the metal legs clacking against each other as they put them on top of their desks and then the tip-tip sound their shoes make as all the kids leave the room.

The teacher is behind me, and coming close to me he breathes, 'And what are we going to do with you, missy, hmm? You've been a very naughty girl again and I'm afraid you are going to have to be punished.'

He turns me around and I am mesmerised to see that he is only wearing his black cloak, socks and shoes. I start to laugh. 'Put out your hand!' he explodes. I do so and he brings a heavy ruler down on my hand with a smack. My eyes start to water, but I don't cry. Instead I hold out my other hand, even though he hasn't told me to. He smacks me again.

'I think it's going to have to be the bottom this time,' he says, 'because you have been a very, very naughty girl.'

He puts me over his knee and starts to spank me very hard. That is all I can remember of the dream.

ANALYSIS
A teacher in a dream represents authority. Lynn is back in a classroom, and judging by the sound of it she is back at primary school. The presence of a school in her dream

suggests that she is still not mature, despite her age. She is afraid to make decisions, which may well be because of the dominant influence that her father had on her from an early age. The classroom could also indicate her current feeling that she would like to do something else as a career. It may be that she will have to go back to study in order to do so.

The corporal punishment inflicted on Lynn means that at present her life is not going too well. On the other hand, now that she has paid the price, her future looks bright. She must now consider her future carefully before making any changes.

CUNNILINGUS

Rachel has been married to Peter, a factory manager who has just celebrated his 40th birthday, for 18 years. They have no children. Theirs is a very traditional marriage: Peter is a chauvinist and while he firmly believes that a wife's place is in the home, Rachel does go out to work.

However, she is expected to keep the house in order, even down to ironing her husband's socks. Peter never praises Rachel publicly when they give dinner to their friends, but instead is very critical. She hides her hurt about this very well. In the bedroom theirs is a very predictable sex life. This is an account of Rachel's dream.

THE DREAM

I am lying naked on an altar and all around me there are men with hoods that cover their faces. I hear a kind of low humming and chanting of music. Looking frantically around me, I am terrified. After muttering what sounds like a Latin hymn over me, the tallest of the men moves forward and produces a knife.

My breath stops and I struggle against the bonds, but when he brings the blade of the knife close to my wrists, he cuts my bonds. Four of the men approach the side of the white-marble altar and with natural sponges and golden bowls of water, they proceed to wash me all over and dab the sweetest-smelling perfume behind my neck, on my breasts, in my navel and behind my knees.

Then, taking turns, they kiss me along my body, ending at my vagina, where each one teases my clitoris with the tip of his tongue. They worship me in this way for ages.

ANALYSIS

Poor Rachel is neglected and taken for granted by her husband. She has sacrificed her life to a very selfish man — hence the appearance of the altar in her dream. However, things take a turn for the better when, instead of being a victim, she becomes the object of adoration. Peter probably never performs cunnilingus on his wife and to have adoring males interested only in giving her pleasure is a revelation for Rachel.

She really should stop being so cosy and dependable and start making some demands on her husband, otherwise she will always be a dogsbody.

DATING

Charlotte recently finished her university exams and although she did not do as well as she had hoped, she passed them all. A plump girl just turned 21, she has had boyfriends but preferred to concentrate on her studies.

The middle child of three sisters, Charlotte was always considered the intelligent one in the family. She remembers her mother trotting out a well-worn phrase throughout her childhood as she patted her on the head: 'You got the brains; those two got the beauty.'

'I'm sure she didn't mean any harm when she said that,' says Charlotte of her mother's thoughtless remark.

Charlotte feels as though she has run out of steam. She is tired and listless and can't see anything good about herself. One of her sisters is a model and the other is married to a man who adores her. 'My brains didn't amount to very much,' she says miserably.

THE DREAM

Standing at a bus-stop I see a guy I know from college. We only know each other on a 'hello' basis, and I have never really spoken to him. Tim belongs to a very trendy set of people — all beautiful, of course. When the bus comes, there is a scramble to get on board and in the mêlée I get pushed against the shelter, and my books catapult out from under my arms and fall open into a dirty puddle.

Tim bends down to help me pick the books up and shakes off the rivulets of grimy liquid that stain the white pages. He grimaces and says, 'Bad luck.' It's then that I really notice him. He has the most azure-blue eyes I have ever seen, framed in glossy black lashes. By this stage my own eyes are watery and I know that I have an ugly face that you get just as you are about to howl.

He sees that I am distressed and says, 'You could do with a nice mug of coffee,' and taking my arm he steers me towards a café a few yards from the bus-stop. The windows of the café are steamed up and when we open the door to go in, the smell of fried food blasts out on to the street, taking my breath away.

We sit at a yellow-speckled melamine table which is covered in tiny grains of white sugar, and he orders drinks from a huge, waxen-faced man standing behind the grubby glass counter.

Then suddenly the scene changes and we are somewhere else, in another restaurant and Tim is holding my left hand, stroking my fingers. He only has eyes for me and looking at him I feel very attracted to him. 'I'm glad you agreed to come out with me,' he says as he takes me on to a tiny dance floor and holds me close to him like they did in the old forties movies.

ANALYSIS

Charlotte was brought up to believe that her best talents were academic. She was conditioned from an early age to accept that she was not pretty. Now, with what she believes to be her failure in the only thing she was ever good at, she feels worthless.

Dreaming about a date with someone you are attracted to reveals that you are feeling unattractive and unwanted yourself. Tim paying her attention as though she was the most beautiful woman he had ever seen boosts her ego and in her wishful way validates her as a person.

Charlotte really ought to look to the future and reinvent herself as someone she really likes. Since her weight makes her feel uncomfortable, she could start a diet to banish her plumpness, and perhaps she could also look at ways of improving her hair and enhancing her features to increase her self-esteem.

DIRTY DANCING

Susan has been working as a TV researcher for the past four months. At 24 she hopes that her next career move will mean she is promoted to producer. She has no shortage of boyfriends and in fact often has to turn down dates. Her immediate boss is a handsome man in his late forties and someone she admires greatly. Lately she finds herself feeling a thrill of excitement whenever he compliments her on a job well done, but theirs has only ever been a business relationship.

Susan's dream was about her boss.

THE DREAM

I walk into a ballroom wearing a stunning clinging dress that shows off my figure. I look like Elle McPherson, the supermodel, and as I walk in people turn to look at me and I hear them asking, 'Who's that?' and others answering, saying, 'That's Susan — she's a producer.'

My hair is a golden blonde and flows down my back over the gold-satin slip dress I am wearing. My boss — let's call him Phil — turns around, and on seeing me his eyes widen and he pushes through the crowd to join me. He asks me to dance and for a while we dance in a very formal way. We chat about work and he tells me he thinks I have a great future ahead of me and that I will climb to the top. When he says that I feel a real glow of pride.

After a dance we part. He says he has to mingle. I can understand that and I too find some people to chat to. But every now and then I catch his eye across the room. As the evening wears on, the room gets hot and eventually I walk out through french windows on to a balcony. Some slow music comes on and suddenly in the doorway, Phil appears, saying, 'May I have the pleasure?' as the sounds of 'Je t'aime' can be heard.

He pulls me towards him and within seconds he is running his hands over my body. The satin against my skin seems to drive him wild, especially as I am not wearing any underwear. He holds me tight against his body. I can feel every part of him against me and soon it seems as though we are merging together until we are one person.

Then suddenly I am looking at myself and it's as though I am a ghost and I have disappeared into his body.

ANALYSIS

Susan is fiercely ambitious and hard-working, and the references to gold (the hair and the satin dress) show that, like any modern working female, she wants to enjoy the financial rewards of her efforts. Flowing hair could indicate an impatience to climb the career ladder — she wants the freedom to go where she thinks she should. Satin is a fabric that can only be worn with confidence, especially when it is as clinging as Susan's dress. It indicates her confidence in herself.

The dancing could be symbolic of many things. Perhaps Susan has a deep longing to be more than just a good professional colleague. Maybe she wants more than praise for her work from Phil. Dancing in a dream often indicates the onset of romance and lovemaking.

DOGGY-FASHION

Marie is a 35-year-old single woman who works in a book-shop. She has been there for seven years and feels as though life is passing her by. She is rarely successful in relationships as she finds it hard to communicate and has never met anybody she feels she would like to spend her life with. She has had two sexual relationships, against her better judgement and her religious beliefs. She is a Catholic, and although she does not practise her faith actively, she does manage to retain the guilt that is some-times associated with the religion.

THE DREAM

I am in the bookshop when a man comes in, the bell on the door announcing his entrance. He is tall with dark good looks and he smiles as he passes the counter. 'Just browsing,' he says. I tell him to help himself. We are the only ones in the shop, it's wet and windy outside and peo-ple are walking past the window, their heads bowed against the weather.

I sigh because I just hate days like this — they just drag on and on until it gets dark at about 3.30 p.m., then I have got feeding the cat to look forward to and a night in front of the TV.

I am pricing some books and the only sound you can hear is the clicking of the pricing machine as I mark each one. I can't see the man but I can hear him taking books from the shelf before looking at them and replacing them.

Damn, I think, as the price tape runs out and I bend behind the desk to look for a refill. It's such a mess down there that I can't find anything. There is a box of hardback books on the floor and I struggle to pull them out from behind the counter so that I can get to the shelf. I am grunting with the effort and not making much progress when I hear him behind me.

'Do you need a hand?' he says, his voice sounding like melting chocolate. Before I can say anything I feel his hands either side of my hips and he is pulling as though to help pull the box. The heat of his palms comes through the cotton dress I am wearing and I shiver.

He runs his palms down the side of my hips, along my legs, until he finds the tops of my stockings. 'Mmm, stockings. Who would have believed it?' he says. When he lifts up my dress I don't move, but I am not scared. He puts his finger under the elastic in my knickers and lazily runs it around the outline before suddenly yanking them down around my ankles.

Then he spreads my legs; I feel the warmth of his skin on mine as he enters me and, leaning across me doggy - fashion, has sex. His whole body is curved to fit mine and he pumps into me relentlessly until with a shudder he empties himself into me.

He withdraws and pulls up my panties, then pulls my dress back down over my bottom before saying, 'Thank you' and leaving. I hear the bell on the door as he opens, then shuts it, and that's where the dream ends.

ANALYSIS
Marie needs a little excitement in her life, but she is waiting for it to come to her. The only place she will get it is in her dreams, and even then she will remain a passive sexual partner..

The fact that she has sex doggy-fashion in her dream says much about Marie's approach to life. She has the potential to live a life that excites her far more — for where did such an exciting dream originate if not within her? But her passions are under tight control and until such time as she stops living within her self-imposed barriers, her life will remain mundane.

DRESSING UP

James and Pippa have been 'an item' for eight months. He fell in love with her when they met at a sales executives' conference. They work for the same company in the computer business. Pippa is a very attractive redhead who has an easy charm with people. Men flock to her side, becoming animated when she talks. She is held in high esteem by her bosses and accordingly has some very prestigious accounts in her portfolio.

James is also good at his job, although sales have been rather slack lately. He is very aware that Pippa enjoys a more powerful position within the company. As a result for the past few months she has been sent abroad by the company to represent them in their bid to expand their markets. This has meant that they have been separated for several days at a time.

James feels threatened by this development and now whenever they meet up, they always seem to have silly rows. However, they make up quickly, although James inevitably feels as if the rows are his fault and lately he is left with a feeling of resentment towards Pippa.

He had the following dream.

THE DREAM

Walking into my bedroom, I go to the wardrobe where Pippa stores her clothes. As I open the door I breathe in deeply, savouring the faint smell of perfume that still lingers on the garments hanging there.

I leave the door ajar and undress slowly, looking at myself in the mirror as I do so. I drop my clothes — a smart suit — where I stand.

The dream jumps and the next thing I am standing in front of the mirror wearing one of her black, short-skirted suits. I look ridiculous and even as I stand there with my big, knobbly knees jutting out below the skirt I know that I look stupid. But I don't take the clothes off and instead I search in the wardrobe for some shoes to wear.

Finding a pair with high heels, I slip them on, and strangely they fit. Then I wobble to the bathroom, where I wash my face, and then I start to brush my teeth. As I do so, I am scrubbing vigorously to get them really clean. When I am finished I smile back into the mirror at my perfect smile, then return to the bedroom.

The lining of the skirt makes a swish-swish sound as I walk and the silky fabric rubs against my manhood, causing me to have an erection. By the time I stand in front of the mirror in the bedroom, I am feeling very pleased with myself.

As I drape myself on the bed in front of the mirror to admire my looks, I smile. But to my absolute horror, my teeth have huge cracks in them and as I watch they crumble into my mouth in tiny pieces. I can feel them rattling around like broken bits of china.

When I woke I had a dreadful sense of unease.

ANALYSIS

Dressing in clothing of the opposite sex usually indicates a sense of conflict within a relationship. For a man to wear his lover's clothes reveals jealousy towards that person. The colour is also important — in this case black. This is a brooding colour synonymous with death and evil. James's negative feelings towards Pippa are evident.

Dressing up in this way is a common enough theme in dreams and it should not be taken at face value. It does not necessarily mean that James is a transvestite or that he has latent gay tendencies. He is jealous of his girl-friend's success at work and that is something that he must deal with if their relationship is going to work. His confidence has taken a bruising, but he is the only one who can restore his sense of self-esteem because the problem stems from within himself.

ENEMAS

Kirsty, 25, has been a very talented singer all her life — it just comes naturally to her. She has never sought to capitalise on her abilities, but recently she sang at a friend's wedding to great acclaim and was invited by a fellow-guest to sing with his band.

Although she was secretly pleased, she decided that she wouldn't take him up on the offer. 'I didn't think I could face an audience night after night. What if they didn't like me?' she says by way of explanation.

It is a month since Kirsty had the offer and in retrospect she now wishes she had the courage to give a singing career a go. Sitting at her desk in the office where she works as a computer programmer, she finds her thoughts punctuated again and again with phrases like 'if only' and 'what if'.

THE DREAM

I am a little girl dressed in a pretty pink frock with matching ankle socks and patent shoes. I am at a big birthday party, and there is lots of lovely food laid out on tables in a sunny garden. It's warm so I suppose it must be summer.

Kids run around playing hide-and-seek and musical chairs, all the time screaming and giggling. I feel happy and I am smiling.

I hear an adult shouting, 'Come on, kids' as another carries out a huge white birthday cake festooned with ribbon and pink icing roses. The top is ablaze with candles and someone in the garden starts up an out-of-tune 'Happy Birthday To You'. Soon everybody is singing along as a blonde-haired girl grins from ear to ear and, puckering up her lips, huffs herself up to blow the flames out.

It takes her a few attempts and we all cheer afterwards. Then someone behind me prods me in the back, pushing me forwards, and says, 'Sing, Kirsty.'

I can feel the atmosphere change and I become very frightened as all the other children start chanting, 'We want Kirsty' over and over again. Then suddenly I faint.

When I wake I am in a hospital bed and a nurse is performing an enema on me. I try to tell them that there is nothing wrong with me but every time I attempt to speak my voice just comes out as a strangled gurgle. The dream ends then.

ANALYSIS

Celebrating a birthday could indicate that deep down Kirsty is celebrating a part of herself that has just been born — the realisation that she has a unique talent that others would pay to hear. But her lack of confidence is holding her back.

Enemas in a dream, although very unpleasant, are a positive sign. She is symbolically being liberated from her worries and inhibitions, purged of her self-inflicted repression and negativity.

Perhaps she should draw inspiration from the words of the poet Goethe, who wrote:

Whatever you can do, or dream you can, begin it. Boldness has genius, power and magic in it.

EROTIC ART

Kieron and Kate have been married for ten years. For the past year they have been trying to have children. When they decided to have a family, Kate came off the pill straight away. Like her husband she is 33, and had taken the contraceptive since she was 17.

'I didn't expect to get pregnant straight away, but I would have thought that surely after one year the effects of the drug on my body would have worn off.'

The pressure to have a child quickly as Kate's biological clock is ticking away is causing great anxiety between the couple. Kieron has said that he feels as though sex has become a chore since the spontaneity of lovemaking has vanished. He has begun to have performance problems.

Kate had the following dream.

THE DREAM

I am in the National Gallery in London on a rainy afternoon. There aren't many people around and I am enjoying my amble through the quiet halls. I walk from one section to another, stopping to stare at Van Gogh's Sunflowers. The colours are really intense and I feel as though I can touch the flowers, they look so real.

As I leave the huge room where that painting is on display, I turn right into a corridor at the end of which I can see some sculptures under a high-ceilinged domed roof. The room seems unusually bright.

Walking down the corridor towards the entrance, I notice that there are no people in the room. When I enter I am astonished to see that every picture on the wall depicts erotic scenes. I feel a little embarrassed and I look around to see if anybody is watching me.

After a little while I relax and sit on one of the long polished wooden benches that are strategically positioned in the room. Like the sunflower painting they also look very real and it seems as if the people in the pictures are three-dimensional. There is an orgy scene with more than a dozen bodies writhing in passion.

Another painting shows a very well-endowed man leaning against a tree as a young woman performs fellatio on him. Everywhere I look there are paintings of sex scenes. I enjoy looking at them and feel very tempted to touch the paint, feel the texture of their passion.

One picture shows a man who looks particularly proud of his manhood as he bends to kiss a naked woman who has her hand clasped around it. I stand in front of the painting and then, looking furtively over my shoulder, I reach up to touch his erection. It is smooth and I imagine it feels real as I run my fingers along its length.

ANALYSIS

It is a particularly difficult time for Kate at the moment. It is obvious that her obsession with having a baby is causing stress and that is not the most conducive thing to creating a good atmosphere in the bedroom. Kate's dream reflects this pressure.

She is standing looking at a collection of erotic art and in a way she is distracting herself from the reality of her situation by watching other people get on with their lives.

The dominant presence of a phallus in her dream indicates her obsession with creativity — in this case, creating a baby.

What she can draw from a dream like this is inspiration. Instead of turning her love-life into a production line, she should bring back a little more spice so that she and Kieron can rekindle the spark that initially set them alight with passion.

EXHIBITIONISM

Mark is a postman, handsome in a cheeky-chap way, and has a great way with women. They love his banter and uninvited compliments as he does his rounds. At 25 he is fit, his body toned from the hours he spends in the gym. He is justifiably proud of it and whenever the weather is good he takes off to the beach to pose.

His steady girlfriend laughs at his obsession with his 'pecs' and he feels that she doesn't realise how important his body is to him. Other women, however, often comment on how good he looks.

THE DREAM

There is a park near the route I take. It is very big and wooded, backing onto a very up-market area. Women take their dogs there for walks at all times during the day; it is very popular.

Inside the park there is a fish sculpture fountain at a point where all the pathways meet. People sit on the benches surrounding it to chat. At the time I go through there are mainly women on the seats.

In my dream I am walking along a path. It's a wonderful sunny day, beautiful blue sky. As I pass two women in their 40s at the fountain, one says, 'Hello, gorgeous.' I stop in my tracks, amazed at how forward she is and she says, 'You are, you know, with that beautiful body.'

As I look down I see my shabby blue and red uniform and my hands move to the buttons. 'You ain't seen nothing yet,' I say as I undo my jacket, then my shirt. Pretty soon I have performed a strip for the ever-increasing audience of women until I am standing there in all my glory.

The women move towards me marvelling at my contours and stroking my muscles as I flex them individually. 'He's like a marble sculpture — Adonis,' says one. 'Yes,' agrees another. 'Wouldn't he be a sight for sore eyes first thing in the morning, instead of that silly fish sculpture?' she says, looking at the fountain.

Suddenly I find myself knee deep in water as I wrestle the fish sculpture from its stand. It's thirsty work and I cup my hands together to take a drink from the spouting tap. Then, climbing on to the pedestal, I stand there with my hands on my hips, flexing my muscles in turn like an international body-builder on stage.

The women clap and whistle and I enjoy all the attention.

But all of a sudden I feel myself start to harden and I can't move my limbs any more; they feel like lead and I can feel my facial movements freeze, my mouth open with surprise. Even though I can't move, I can still see people looking at me, then the crowd parts and my girlfriend is standing there shaking her head and saying 'What a silly man.' Then the dream ends.

ANALYSIS

Mark's obsession with his body is overwhelming, as his dream indicates, and bordering on the unhealthy. He must realise that the cliché 'beauty is only skin deep' is true if you concentrate solely on your physical appearance. But what he may not realise is that his obsession is driving his girlfriend away from him and that she may find it utterly boring that their everyday conversations revolve around his physique.

The dream suggests a man who is not really at ease with himself, and the need for adulation by the women in the park as he displays himself shows that. Drinking water from a fountain, although done purely to quench his thirst in his dream, can also represent him drinking in all the sexual adulation and could mean that he is quenching his sexual desires.

The petrification of Mark's body into stone show a deadness in the spirit of his relationship with his girl-friend, and her arrival at the end of the dream endorses this interpretation.

FLAGELLATION

Twenty-four-year-old Louise is a student. An only girl, she was the apple of her father's eye. He was so possessive of her that when she grew into a pretty teenager he actively discouraged her from going out with boys. When she was 18 and had left home for university she fell in love with a fellow-student.

He was the first person Louise had ever slept with, and she got pregnant. Desperate that her father should not find out, she arranged to have a secret abortion. He would have been horrified if he had known what had happened to his daughter. He never did.

Louise had her dream during the week of her father's funeral. His death hit her particularly hard because she was away when he had a fatal heart attack. 'I find it very difficult to come to terms with because I never got a chance to say goodbye,' she says.

THE DREAM

I am taken walking down a long corridor of what seems to be a convent or monastery. The flagstones are cool beneath my naked feet as I pad along silently. Long shadows are cast across the whitewashed walls as the sun sets. Open doors along the corridor let shafts of sunlight fall on to the floor.

It is very peaceful and quiet, but I feel very heavy-hearted. I seem to be wearing a loose shift in a creamy colour and my hair is long like it was when I was 18. As I come to the last door, I knock and a voice tells me to come in. It is a man's voice and when I hear it I really don't want to go into the room. As I hesitate outside the door, the man says, 'I told you to come in now !'

I jump with fright and as I hold the handle down the door creaks open. He is standing leaning on both hands behind a table with two other people, one either side of him. It is like a court scene.

Then the dream seems to jump because suddenly I hear him say, 'Guilty.' The word echoes round and round in my head, but I'm confused. What am I guilty of? Before I have a chance to say anything two policemen take me by the arms and while one holds me the other takes off my shift. Then, like something out of a medieval scene, a masked torturer walks towards me swishing a whip that looks like a bunch of snakes. He smiles and cracks it against the ground before trailing it across my trembling body, over my breasts and down between my legs. It tickles my skin in an awful way and I can feel my flesh crawl.

He continues doing this in the middle of the room and there are a hundred eyes looking at me as if I am a prize exhibit. Then, just as he raises the whip above his head as if to strike me, the crowd chant, 'Guilty, guilty.'

I woke up with a start and my heart was pounding.

ANALYSIS

Louise is punishing herself for what she believes she has done wrong: her abortion and the fact she was not there to say goodbye to her father. Whips are always an unfavourable sign in a dream because inevitably the scourging is self-inflicted.

Louise must learn to let go of the past and forgive herself. She should be proud of her achievements and realise that she must make decisions that will make her happy.

FOOD

Food has always been a problem for Antonella, who at the age of 32 has spent most of her life battling against the bulge. As a child she was known as Fatty by other cruel children. It's a battle she has failed to win — until now. A drastic combination of bingeing and vomiting has ensured that she has been her thinnest for years.

'I have the same disease Princess Diana had: bulimia. I know it is deeply damaging but I can't seem to stop. Like my eating habits, I swing from one end of an emotional pendulum, which is sheer joy, through to the darkest depressions.'

She recently watched a video of the hit movie *9½ Weeks* and marvelled at the food scene where Kim Basinger is fed by Micky Rourke while she wears a blindfold in a prelude to one of Hollywood's hottest sex scenes.

The idea that food could be sexy was anathema to Antonella, but instead of taking a positive message from the film all she did was gorge and make herself sick after watching it.

'I was probably more interested in how thin Kim was,' she says.

THE DREAM

About a week after I saw that film I had a dream in which I saw myself playing Kim Basinger's part as she tasted all the foods offered to her. Even though I looked like Kim in my dream, and even had her body, I knew it was me on the kitchen floor by the fridge and not really her.

The dream then shifted and I couldn't really see much

except a hand coming towards me through a chink in the blindfold. It was holding a spoon and a voice said, 'Come on now, open wide.' I remember hesitating and then opening my mouth and a spoon was shoved in, hitting off the front of my teeth.

It was something warm and meaty and I chewed on it although it was really very soft and liquid. Then, before I had a chance to swallow it, the voice said, 'Open wide, there's a good little girl.'

When I refused to obey, the person said, 'Well then, no dessert for you.' It is at that point that I lift up my blindfold and come face to face, not with Micky Rourke, but with my mother, who is sitting there tut-tutting at me.

'You'll never grow up to be a big girl if you don't eat. Mummy is very upset with you.'

I open my mouth as she shovels huge spoonfuls of the brown stew into my mouth and then goes on to feed me babies' puréed apple from a small glass jar as it dribbles off my chin and on to a bib. That's where the dream ends.

ANALYSIS

Food in dreams suggests a need for nourishment. It may not necessarily be a physical need for food, but rather a desire for emotional satisfaction. It is significant that what is essentially an erotic situation results in Antonella's being spoonfed by her mother.

Her relationship with her mother is the key to Antonella's obsession with food and her appearance. The pressure to 'eat up' that she experienced as a young child has resulted in her developing a negative outlook to her diet and to food in general.

The presence of baby food indicates that Antonella

should 'grow up' and take responsibility for herself by accepting her body for what it is. She needs to seek professional help to beat her disease.

GANG-BANG

Louise is a 29-year-old teacher in a secondary school. She teaches food technology, a job she loves. As a child she loved to cook and make clothes. She didn't inherit her abilities from her mother, who always cremated anything she cooked and couldn't sew on a button.

But Louise had a natural aptitude for what was essentially home-making. Teaching was one way of making her skill pay its way. There were days when she didn't look forward to going to work, and like anybody she experienced the Monday blues, but lately she had begun to feel like she didn't fit in at work.

Louise's feelings coincided with the arrival of a new head of department who very quickly made it clear that she thought very little of her teaching ability. Clearly she felt that Louise's unorthodox method of letting the kids have a free run of the class was not in keeping with her standards. As a result, there followed what seems to have been a whispering campaign, and more often than not Louise found that conversation suddenly stopped when she joined her colleagues.

Her dream came at a time when she was recovering from a bout of flu, and on the Sunday before she was due back at school to start a new week she had a fitful night.

THE DREAM
The school bell goes and as usual all my pupils make a mad dash for the door. They can't bear to spend a second more than they have to at school. We have been cooking pancakes and the place is a bit of a tip.

The kids have taken it in turns to toss pancakes and unfortunately not everyone managed to catch them with the pan after throwing them in the air. One even hit the ceiling and stuck there.

We all laughed our heads off, even though I know I shouldn't encourage them. I told the young boy who threw it that I would climb on the stepladder and clear off the bits stuck to the ceiling when class was over. I didn't want him to fall and break his neck.

I was wearing a tartan skirt and red polo-neck jumper and a pair of opaque stockings. I wore a pink frilled pinny over my clothes to keep them relatively clean.

Miss Crisp, the new head of department, had taken to turning up after every cookery lesson I took, to check up on me, and I was aware that the place looked like a bomb site. There was flour everywhere.

First I took off my shoes and climbed up the stepladder to clean the ceiling. As I reached up with a cloth and rubbed the mess, I could hear the sounds of the children's voices fade as fewer of them remained in the building.

It was dark and gloomy outside, the grey skies threatening to swamp us again with rain. It matched my mood.

The sports master popped his head around the door with two men I hadn't seen before. He was a new guy himself, not long with the school. I didn't like him because he was really leery.

Before I could scramble down from the ladder, he came over and ran his hand up my leg. I slapped him away and as I lost my balance he grabbed me and, helped by the other two men, he held me down on the ground before ripping my clothes off. There they took turns to have sex with me. I tried to scream but I couldn't — no sound would come.

As I lay there covered in flour I heard the unmistakable sharp click-click of Miss Crisp's shoes in the hallway. She stood in the doorway, a look of revulsion on her face, before she turned and walked away.

I felt a terrible sense of shame and even when I woke it was still with me.

The Monday I was due back to school I just couldn't face going because I felt as if those two teachers would know what had gone on in my dreams the night before.

ANALYSIS

Louise's dream shows that her self-esteem is very low. The presence of a rape scene in a dream is not indicative of a fantasy desire to be raped. Louise is obviously a very gentle person and is allowing Miss Crisp's negativity to rub off on her.

The fact is that while Miss Crisp obviously doesn't like Louise, she has not really interfered with her working day, in that she has not formally criticised her abilities. The reality is that she probably has no real reason to, because the exam results show that Louise's methods of teaching do reap benefits for the pupils.

The presence of a rape scene in the dream shows that negative energy is building up, sapping Louise's power. She should hold her head up high, stand back from the problem and be professional but polite to Miss Crisp. As soon as the head of department knows she cannot bully Louise, she will back down.

GENITALS

Dominic lost his job at a well-known bank last year, one of many redundancies made during a cost-cutting initiative. For the first six months he tried almost daily to get another job, but application after application was met with rejection. He could have got a more menial job but when he and his wife, Sonia, did their sums, they concluded that it would not be financially viable for him to do so.

Sonia also worked as a solicitor. She was dynamic and very respected by her colleagues. The couple have two children, both of school age, and it was while they were very young that Sonia studied to be a solicitor.

The couple discussed their situation and came to the conclusion that it would be better if Dominic stayed at home to look after the children. That way they could dispense with the nanny and save money. It was only going to be a temporary solution and then, as soon as it seemed that the work market had improved, he would try to find another job.

Three months into the arrangement, Dominic was feeling frustrated and angry. Sonia was staying later at the office as she took on more work. She was seizing the opportunity of no longer having to rush home to relieve the childminder of the children, and concentrating on her career instead.

Dominic originally thought it was going to be easy to run a household, but has come to the conclusion he is not very good at it. He finds he has practically nothing to talk to Sonia about any more. To make things worse, he sees no one and feels very lonely.

Dominic had a dream about his situation.

THE DREAM

I am standing in the kitchen watching the washing machine overflow. I am absolutely mesmerised by the way the suds are thick and creamy-looking and multiply at an alarming rate. I don't move, just stand there.

Behind me the kitchen is a mess, food everywhere, un-ironed washing, dishes on the table, an upturned cereal box has spilled its contents on to the kitchen floor and the dog is snuffling round them, licking the bright yellow flakes up with his tongue.

I feel panic rising inside me and I know that I am just not going to be able to cope. The kids are sitting glued to the television, watching some blaring American cartoon series. I know they should really be sitting down reading, but I just can't be bothered to tell them to. Anyway it's less effort if I don't have to entertain them.

Eventually the washing machine rattles to a halt and I step in the bubbles to retrieve the washing. The clothes are still thick with suds, but I just throw them on to the line to dry. As I look over the garden fence I see my wife walking towards me.

Swearing, I dive back into the kitchen, hit the floor and sprain my ankle. As the pain shoots up my leg I'm muttering to myself, 'She's not supposed to be here for at least three hours.'

I hear her keys in the lock and the front door pushes open. As she walks in the kids run out to greet her in the hallway, excited to see her as if she has just returned from a long voyage.

As she stood in the doorway of the kitchen, she looked furious and was about to shout at me when she looked at my face. Tears were streaming down my cheeks.

Helping me to my feet, she supported me as I hobbled

to the bathroom. 'A nice hot bath for you,' she said. 'That'll make you feel better.'

As the bath water ran, filling the room up with steam, I rub a patch in the mirror and look at the dishevelled, lifeless face that stares back. Outside I can hear my wife cleaning up. I know the place will be immaculate when I go out.

I take off my clothes and sit in the hot water, then reach for the soap and rub it across my body, down my stomach and over my genitals — but there is nothing there. My penis and scrotum are gone. I stand up and look down to check, but all I find is a vagina. I start to scream and wake up feeling very jittery.

ANALYSIS

The presence of genitals in any dream is indicative of a creative, reproductive energy. Clearly Dominic feels his current role as house-husband is stemming that creativity. The loss of his penis indicates that he feels emasculated by the mountain of daily chores he faces.

Dominic is not unique in the way he feels, for countless women feel as he does every day and unfortunately for them it is seen as the norm that they should stay at home and look after the kids and the house.

He should take a leaf out of his wife's book and, instead of moping and feeling sorry for himself, he should arrange to further his education, as this will help him to get an even better job. Sonia is taking advantage of him and she must be made to realise that she, too, has a role to play in the home, just as when they both had jobs.

The presence of a fence in the dream indicates that there are hurdles to jump. Dominic could see over it, and this says that with a little bit of effort all their problems will be scaled. In particular, it is important for the couple not to let resentment build up between them.

GOD/GODDESS

Elaine is a very happy person. She recently got the job of her dreams as a presenter on a local radio station, the first stepping stone to the big time. She is in love with a great guy who feels the same way about her.

She gets on well with her parents and her sister Fiona and brother Thomas, who are both younger than her. In all she has very little to complain about.

THE DREAM

There is a carnival and everybody is happy and excited. It seems to be set in somewhere like India – the streets are full of paper streamers and everyone is wearing brightly coloured silks. There's not one person who isn't smiling.

The carnival is in honour of a goddess, and there is a procession winding its way through the throngs of people. Huge floats covered in sweet-smelling yellow and white flowers go past me. I feel deliciously happy.

Suddenly, to the sound of a gong, a very ornate float appears and there is a statue of a beautiful woman with gold-coloured clothes draped over her. As the float draws closer, it stops in front of me and the whole crowd bow towards me.

At first I'm perplexed until I realise that the goddess they are worshipping is me. As they do so, a row of hunky tanned men walk up the platform to where I am sitting on a gold throne and place offerings of fruit, jewels and perfumes at my feet. Then one anoints my forehead, feet and wrists with exotic perfume. The crowd cheer and I smile back at them.

ANALYSIS

This is a very pleasant dream, in which the presence of a goddess (a god has the same significance for a man) indicates that Elaine is very much at ease with herself. The goddess is a powerful positive symbol that radiates love and unity. Elaine obviously has very little to worry about at the moment.

GROPING

Patrick and Bernadette have been together since they were 17. They met at the local disco and within minutes struck up a bond that was to last for seven years. During those years their two families also became very close, even meeting up regularly for Sunday lunch.

When Patrick and Bernadette announced their engagement last year, everyone was naturally thrilled. Their mothers got together immediately to discuss the wedding arrangements.

Unfortunately, instead of cementing Bernadette's happiness, the impending wedding only served to make her feel unsure. Now she feels that the only reason she agreed to get married was because she is trying to please everybody else. Last week, after yet another row with Patrick, she stormed out of his parents' house.

Walking back to her own home just a few roads away, she bumped into one of Patrick's friends, Sean, who had just come back from a trip with the Royal Navy.

It was the first time she had seen him in two years. He seemed delighted to see her and invited her to pop down to the local pub with him for a homecoming drink. She agreed reluctantly at first, but after the second glass of white wine she began to relax, listening to his tales of countries she had never seen and probably never would.

When Sean walked her home to her front door, he kissed her goodnight. It was the first time she had been kissed by another man since she began going out with Patrick. It felt wonderful and she could sense a feeling of excitement rising inside her.

Her mother was waiting for her when she walked into

the living room. Emboldened by the wine, she began to say she was having second thoughts. Her mother told her not to be so ridiculous; she reminded her of the huge sacrifices she and her father were making to help pay for the wedding and, bursting into tears, told her that Bernadette couldn't possibly think of embarrassing her family by calling the wedding off. What would people think?

Then, leaving her daughter sitting on the sofa, she stormed upstairs. To the sound of her parents' agitated conversation in the room above, Bernadette fell asleep.

This is the dream she had that night.

THE DREAM

I am standing having a conversation with my family and Patrick's family. I leave them and walk away, looking back every now and then. They are just standing there looking at me, a pool of light illuminating them.

I feel a sense of freedom as I walk away and move towards a tunnel. As I pass through I feel hands coming from the darkness, touching me and caressing me. I'm not frightened and quite enjoy the new sensation of feeling a stranger's hands on me.

It's a delicious, abandoned feeling, and I revel in it, holding my arms above my head as I let the hands roam over my body. Still moving through the tunnel, I pass along a variety of hands, but suddenly the mood changes.

The movements of the hands become rough and grabbing. I now find myself slapping them away as they are beginning to hurt me and pull me. I hear a rip as the fabric in my dress is torn and I am spun in a circle. I look behind me to see if my family is still waiting for me, but there is no light.

The hands grab me even harder and pull me towards what look like grilles in the wall. I tussle with them and try to break free, but even though I can't see whose hands they are I feel as though they are familiar.

When I wake up, I'm freezing cold and the living room clock says 4 a.m. I get up and go to my bedroom, where I lie awake until it's time to get up for work.

ANALYSIS

Groping in a dream can represent strong emotional attachment. This is its positive aspect, but in some cases it can turn into a claustrophobic attachment. It is obvious from Bernadette's dream that hers is the second.

She feels as though she is being dragged into something that she doesn't really want to get involved in. She needs to set aside some time for herself and really think things through. The decision she makes now is one that will affect her for the rest of her life. There is no point in going along with plans now for a quiet life. She is the one who is going to have to lie in the bed she has made.

It may be that she is just getting a case of jitters, but she needs to sort out her feelings. At this stage, getting involved with another man is definitely not a good idea.

HEROES

Craig has never been much of an action man. At school he shied away from the more robust sports like rugby and football. He was always a loner, preferring to concentrate on his studies rather than mix with the rest of the boys at school. And yet he wasn't short of friends and as he grew older he had no difficulty in finding girlfriends.

Recently he was watching on television a real-life drama in which a man and his child were in an upturned car in a river. They couldn't get out and the water was rising very fast. The man's child was sitting in the back seat of the car, crying.

Eventually, with a huge burst of energy, the man managed to free himself, climb out into the swirling water and break the back window to get to his son.

Craig became very emotional watching this because when he was a child himself a young girl he knew drowned when she was just 12 years old. After that he had never felt safe near water.

THE DREAM
The water is swirling and black and I'm drowning. As I panic I take in huge gulps of air and water at the same time. I hear a voice shouting, 'Help.' It's a woman's voice and I realise that it is me shouting for help.

All of a sudden I shoot out of the water with a woman in my arms. She is limp and lifeless. As I take her out of the water, I hear people clapping and cheering. I am flying with her in my arms above their heads.

I lay the woman on a patch of grass and holding her

mouth open and her nose closed, I gently blow air into her lungs. She coughs and splutters and tries to sit up, but instead I make her lie on her side until she starts to breathe normally.

She looks up at me and I realise she has the bluest eyes I have ever seen. She is gorgeous. Then, as I am looking at her, she reaches up and puts her arms around my shoulders and pulling herself up she whispers, 'My hero,' and kisses me deeply. I feel my head spinning as I drown in her kiss.

A warmth spreads through my body and I feel myself getting turned on. When the kiss stops, people clap and pat me on the back, saying, 'Well done.' I stand up and realise that I am dressed as Superman. Then I tell them I have to go and that's where the dream ends.

ANALYSIS

Craig's dream can be seen as a sort of wish-fulfilment dream. The TV programme triggered off memories that had lain dormant in his subconscious for many years. He was a child when his school chum died and no doubt that terrible experience left him with a sense of helplessness. Real heroes are people who do something out of the ordinary to help others, often putting their own lives at risk.

In his dream Craig was drowning yet he mustered up the courage to save someone else. The presence of Superman in the dream indicates that he wishes to emulate this extraordinary man. But if Craig wants to take any message from this courageous dream, then he should set about overcoming his fear of water, then learn how to swim and how to resuscitate someone. Who knows, maybe some day he really will be a hero.

HOMOSEXUALITY

Peter has known Ralph since he was a young boy. They met at a boarding school where they realised they were virtual neighbours, living only a few streets from each other. As youngsters growing up, they became firm friends, meeting during the long school holidays to play rugby, fish and swim.

Ralph was a confident, articulate boy who charmed adults and his peers alike. A 'thoroughly nice bloke' was a phrase often used to describe him. He was good at practically everything he touched, including both sports and his studies, and when he was a teenager the girls fell for his dark good looks.

The two young men went their separate ways after school, Peter to a redbrick university, and Ralph to Cambridge, like his father before him. During this time they maintained their relationship. It was only when Ralph got engaged to a woman just as successful as he was that Peter started to compare his own life with his friend's. Recently he has found that he was making excuses not to meet up with his old school chum because he felt a failure whenever they met.

Peter had a dream about their relationship.

THE DREAM
Sitting in my living room, I have the lights turned down low, the fire is crackling in the grate and Polly, my Persian cat, is sitting on my lap purring deeply as I languidly stroke her. I am listening to some classical music while I read a book. It's very relaxing.

Suddenly the doorbell goes. As I get up to answer it I am surprised to have a caller at this late stage of the night. In the hall, I can make out the shadow of a man at the door and, looking through the spy-hole, I am surprised to see it is Ralph.

At first I hesitate to open the door. I don't know if I want to let him in or not. But he knows I am there and says, 'Come on, Peter, it's freezing out here.'

He stands on the steps, his shoulders all hunched, a worried look on his face. As he steps in, the hallway gets cold and I usher him into the heat of the living room. He sits on the sofa and I bring him a warming drink of brandy.

He gulps it down in one go and holds the glass out for another one. I top him up. He plays with the rim of his glass, making that squeaking sound you get when the rim is wet, and stares at the flames in the fireplace.

I ask him what is wrong and am horrified to see that his eyes fill with tears. At once I sit beside him and try to coax him to tell me.

'She's gone,' he says finally.

His fiancée, Lesley, had left him. I put my arms around his shoulders and give him what starts out as a brotherly hug, but the next thing I know I am kissing him and he is kissing me back passionately.

The next part of my dream shows us lying on the floor in front of the fire, naked and aroused, caressing each other. But our amorous exploits are interrupted by the sound of Polly miaowing to be allowed out of the room.

That is the sound I wake up to. At first I don't remember the dream and then later on in the morning it comes back to me. I felt revolted at the memory. I have never fancied any man before or even thought of taking my relationship with Ralph any stage further. Is this dream telling me I have hidden sexual urges? I really can't believe it is, but then what is the message it is giving?

ANALYSIS

Homosexual or lesbian activity in a dream does not automatically indicate that you have submerged feelings for the same sex. Homosexuality in dreams refers to the masculine part of a male dreamer (or the feminine part of a female dreamer), so in effect Peter is trying to come to terms with his emotions as a man.

Dreaming that you are having a sexual relationship with someone of the same sex to whom you are close could indicate a wish to have the attributes you admire in that other person. Peter, while proud of Ralph, can't help but feel slightly inadequate in the face of his friend's success.

His closeness to Ralph in the dream merely indicates his wish to be more like him. However, outside the world of dreams, their relationship is hitting a rocky patch. Peter needs to try to think about his own good qualities and to concentrate on them.

ICE QUEEN

Natasha, 29, recently met a new man for whom she feels a great deal of affection but she finds it hard to contemplate a long-term relationship. Her last boyfriend broke her heart. They had been together for five years and she had expected to marry him, for he had always intimated it. She eventually found out that he was two-timing her when her mother spotted him kissing a younger woman.

He had been too cowardly to tell her that their relationship was over and even after her mother saw him, he didn't contact her — she had to find him to ask him what was going on.

THE DREAM

I am at a favourite spot by a lake on a beautiful summer's day. I am with a man and I feel very optimistic and happy. We are eating sandwiches and drinking champagne. Nearby there is a tape recorder playing Madame Butterfly.

The man I am with touches my face and pulling me towards him, kisses me. We kiss many times and I can feel him getting turned on. But when he starts to move his lips along my neck and kisses my shoulders I feel myself stiffen and freeze. The sun goes in and it starts to cloud over and I feel really cold and shivery.

The man I am with says I am like a block of ice. I feel hard and cold towards him and the magic spell of a beautiful summer's day is broken. The man says, 'You are a bit of an ice-queen. Are you frigid or something?'

He gets up and walks away and as he does I notice that the lake is frozen over.

ANALYSIS

In dreams ice is traditionally representative of frigidity or coldness. Natasha's emotions are hard and brittle like ice. She has built a barrier around her and she does not want it to be crossed. But she should not tar all men with the same brush as that of her ex. He was a coward and she should allow people to make their own mistakes. In order to bring about a thaw in her emotions, Natasha should look for the good in the men she meets. Otherwise she is in danger of never letting anyone get close to her again. At the moment she feels like a victim, but if she doesn't let go of the past, that will become a self-fulfilling prophecy.

IMPOTENCE

Frank has reached his forties and he is not feeling too good about it. It is a well-known fact that many men go through a crisis around this time of life.

Recently he was passed over for promotion and a man four years his junior got the job instead. Naturally Frank was very disappointed and can't shake the feeling that his chance has been lost. At his age he feels that time is passing him by and that the way up is blocked for many years to come. He has two main options: either settle down and get on with the job he has or try to move to pastures new.

He has been scanning the appointments pages and although the competition is sure to be tough, there are a number of positions on offer. But he feels as though his confidence has taken a severe blow and is not sure that anyone would really want him.

THE DREAM

I am sitting in front of a panel of interviewers. There are three men and one woman, all quizzing me. Then the woman, who is pretty ordinary-looking, says, 'What about your performance, how does that rate?'

I am a bit taken aback and I start to stutter, saying, 'I think I'm pretty good, I've got a good track record.' Then she turns to the others on the panel and says, 'I think we should have a demonstration.'

They all murmur agreement and it is with a heavy heart that I try to comply. As I step out of my trousers, a woman knocks on the door and enters the room. She is wearing really sexy lingerie with stockings and suspenders. I am standing in front of all of these people with my socks and shoes on and my trousers and boxer shorts down around my ankles, feeling very stressed.

The sexy woman walks over to me and touches my manhood, but there is only a half-hearted response. She then bends down and performs oral sex but to no avail.

The panel look disgusted and start to talk to each other, before one says, 'Next' and throws his pen down on the table. I feel absolutely mortified and the scantily-clad woman flicks her hair and walks off.

ANALYSIS

Frank has a severe case of self doubt. Dreaming of not being able to perform sexually is related to the anxiety he feels during the day. He has got his being passed over for promotion completely out of proportion. It happens all the time and often it is not because the candidate is unable to do the job, but a question of office politics.

It would boost Frank's confidence greatly if he applied for some of those jobs. If nothing else they will show him just how far he can get on his own merits. Then he will open up options for himself. But he must do it sooner rather than later because the longer he leaves it the greater the problem will become.

INCEST

Penny has never really felt close to her parents, who are not demonstrative people. An only child, she always felt as though she was in the way and they didn't really want her around. She tried hard to please them, studied conscientiously at school to achieve good results and never gave them cause to scold her if she could avoid it. In short her entire life was spent trying to please her parents.

Even when she managed to get a good job in a bank and work her way up to be an assistant manager, they never seemed proud and happy for her. Penny feels a little silly that at her age, now 33, she should still feel hurt by her parents' reactions.

THE DREAM

I see a little girl with a pretty dress skipping down a path and I feel compelled to follow her to see where she is going. I can't see her face but I know from the way she is skipping that she is happy.

She comes to a huge house and pushes open a heavy door, which creaks closed behind her just as I come up the path. I hear her shout, 'Mummy, Daddy.' I stand there looking at the closed door and then I hear the sound of footsteps as she goes down to the basement kitchen.

I walk past a huge bush, feeling compelled to look in the window to see what she is doing. As I do so I am horrified when I see a man whose face I can't see undoing her pretty little dress. It falls to the floor and she is standing there in a white vest and matching knickers.

He takes off her underwear and at first I think he is

going to wash her, but even in my dream I realise that is incongruous as she is in the kitchen. The little girl has her back to me and she is trembling. The man reaches his hand up and starts to run it over the girl's body.

With a shock I realise he is indecently assaulting her and involuntarily I bang on the window. The man jumps away from the little girl. They both look up at me and I get an even bigger shock when I realise that the little girl is me, and that through her tear-stained face she looks grateful.

It was the weirdest dream because I know that I was not abused as a child.

ANALYSIS

Most dreams represent different aspects of oneself. Often when we dream of seeing someone doing something, then it really is the dreamer who is carrying out the act.

Dreams of incest that are not based on reality or a history of abuse are not dreams of wish-fulfilment; they do not mean that you want to have sex with either your mother or your father. In fact they are dreams where you are integrating the two parts of yourself, namely the adult and the child.

In the dream Penny stopped the abuse the little girl was suffering, and similarly she can stop the hurt she is feeling in her adult life. Penny needs to love herself before others can love her, she needs to realise that if she waits passively for her parents to break the rule of a lifetime by acknowledging her achievements, then she will always be miserable.

Perhaps she would feel better if she could confront them with her feelings. However, she should only do so if she feels that she is strong enough to cope with their inevitable denials.

INFIDELITY

Alison has been friends with Emma for so many years she can scarcely remember how long. So when Emma got herself a new boyfriend, Alison was a little bit jealous. She didn't want to have to share her friend's affection and she knew that it would mean they would spend less time with each other.

She wasn't prepared to like Emma's boyfriend, Chris, but when she met him she immediately realised what her friend saw in the man. After a few months she found that she looked forward to seeing him and he seemed to like her a lot and they always bantered with each other.

Emma told Alison that she was pleased that she and Chris were getting on so well. Alison felt a twinge of guilt when she realised that she felt more for Chris than just friendship and she thought that he was beginning to feel the same.

THE DREAM

I am at a party which is for Emma and Chris's engagement party. As I walk down the stairs, Chris is coming up. I had been to the bathroom, where I had spent time trying to control myself not to cry in public. I felt a great sense of loss and deep misery.

When I saw Chris, he smiled at me and asked me if I was enjoying myself. I forced a smile, but he seemed to sense that something was up. He patted me on the face and as he did so tears spilled down my cheeks. Within a second he was kissing me and caressing me. I remember feeling very nervous at that time.

In the next part of the dream I was in a strange bedroom passionately kissing a man who I think was Chris. He had his hands on the top of my stockings when I heard my name being called.

I pushed him away and took off running, down the stairs, past the front door and out into the street. It seemed as if I was running for ages as my legs started to feel like lead.

ANALYSIS

If Alison values Emma's friendship, she will take this dream as a warning to steer clear of Chris. Dreams of infidelity or adultery are portents of distress and unhappiness. She needs to stop running and face her emotions.

She can do one of two things. She can either talk to Chris about how she feels — after all, she seems to think that he harbours the same thoughts about her. But is she prepared to lose Alison's friendship over a relationship that may or may not work? Or she can try to make new friends so that she doesn't have to see Alison and Chris so much. That way, in time she will find someone who is right for her and her feelings for Chris will change.

JEALOUSY

Jeanine has a friend she can't bear to see. Every time they meet up, something great seems to have happened in her life and she always looks great. While Jeanine battles with a weight problem and always seems to have a crop of spots, Clare exudes radiance. She knows that two people really can't be expected to be the same, but nevertheless she has started to resent Clare's good fortune.

Jeanine has started to make bitchy comments about Clare to other friends. However, whenever Clare phones her to arrange to meet up, she feels compelled to go. It is as though she has to get the next stage in the story of her friend's life.

THE DREAM
I am at a party, it's really great, the music is good and the company even better. I am with my friend — I don't know if it is Clare but I feel as though it is her. We are dancing away and I look great, slim and vivacious. My friend nudges me and points to a really good-looking guy who is leaning against a door frame drinking beer from a bottle. 'He's mine,' she says. He catches my eye and comes over. My friend thinks he is coming to talk to her but he ignores her and talks to me. She is furious and when he asks me to dance I can see that she is really jealous.

The guy 's name is Kevin and we end up spending the whole party together, snogging and smooching to the slow songs. At the end he asks me if he can take me home and I say yes. My friend has already flounced off in a huff, but I really don't care.

ANALYSIS

As in waking life, jealousy is a very negative emotion. Jealousy in dreams may be a case of straightforward wish-fulfilment. If someone in your dreams is jealous of you, then it reflects your own insecurity about your own self worth and that is a problem that it is necessary to address.

Jeanine should make the best of the qualities she has and not focus on what others have got. She needs to re-evaluate the friendship with Clare and really look at what they are both getting out of it. If the negative emotions continue, she should consider ending the relationship.

JEWELLERY

Tony has been with his girlfriend for four years. They met at college. She is studying to be a doctor, while he is a lawyer. He has found himself a job with a reputable firm which he really enjoys. Helen wants to go on to study surgery. She has been offered the opportunity to travel to the USA, where she can continue her studies and be in a position to take her pick of the jobs when she graduates.

This is causing a lot of friction between the couple. Helen has said that she wants Tony to go with her, but he feels settled in London and doesn't see why she can't continue on with her studies there. She on the other hand says he is being sexist and she doesn't see any reason for him not following her to America.

Tony feels that Helen may not love him the way she used to. He had the following dream.

THE DREAM

I am in a room, turning it upside down as I look for something. I keep muttering, 'They were here, I'm sure they were.' My girlfriend is with me and she's crying saying, 'It's such bad luck. What are we going to do?'

I am feeling exhausted as I turn everything over and over again. I hug my girlfriend and tell her that everything will be all right. 'But will it?' she says.

We hug closely and I kiss the top of her head. Then out of the corner of my eye I see a glint just under a box. I feel excitement mount and I race over to the box. On lifting it up I find the necklace we had lost. It's a spectacular thing like something that Princess Di would wear., with huge, sparkly diamonds and three emeralds in a row.

My girlfriend stands while I put it around her neck and fix the clasp. She spins around and kisses me and we fall back on to the sofa in the middle of the churned-up room. We kiss passionately and she starts to take her clothes off.

ANALYSIS

The presence of jewels in a dream does not necessarily denote riches of a material kind. In this dream they represent something that Tony feels he has lost — the love of his girlfriend. By looking for the jewels he is trying to find the love he believes he has lost. But in his waking life Tony is confusing the issues. His girlfriend is not saying she no longer loves him, but that she has to move on with her life and, having spent so many years studying, she should be allowed to reap the rewards.

Tony should have faith in their relationship, for diamonds in a dream denote eternity and life, while emeralds represent faithfulness and hope. Perhaps they should consider Helen going on her own for a while to see how things work out. Whatever they decide to do, Tony should take the dream as a good omen.

JOKER

Geoff is a very quiet person, and would never stand out in a crowd. In fact he would hate to do so. Ironically, he is very attracted to a young woman who works in the office of his firm of architects. She is very sexy and she knows it. Sylvia is a terrible flirt with all the guys and she gives them a really hard time. They all fancy her and would love to date her, but she keeps them at arm's length.

But when it comes to Geoff she treats him as though he were a little kid and she is gentle with him, as though she knows that he couldn't take the ribbing like the other guys or – as Geoff is prone to thinking – she might even fancy him. But he hasn't got the courage to ask her out.

THE DREAM

I am getting ready for a date. As I dress I sing and I feel very happy. After I splash a final bit of aftershave on I leave my room.

The next scene has me waiting for a bus to go into town. It's cold and blustery and I pull my coat around me to keep the chill out.

I am on my way to the pictures, where I am going to meet my date. I get off the bus two stops early because I have given myself too much time to get there and I don't want to appear uncool by looking too eager.

As I near the cinema I see a group of people standing stamping from one foot to another to try to keep warm. To the left of them is another group of people who are very loud and jocular; surrounding somebody who is dressed in a joker's outfit. Probably collecting for charity, I think.

105

But on coming closer I realise that the joker is in fact my date and surrounding her are some of my work colleagues. I also realise the joker is Sylvia. I feel an intense sense of disappointment and feel very foolish. She prances around me, bells jingling and tinkling, and I can hear her laughing.

ANALYSIS

There is an old saying, 'Many a true word is said in jest.' Sylvia's jocular behaviour at work is reflected in the dream although it is taken to greater heights with the presence of the joker figure. The dream is warning Geoff to take heed of his instincts by remaining just colleagues with Sylvia. If she is as flighty as he describes her, then she will always be on the lookout for the next person in her life.

He could become friends with her, but she sounds far too immature for him to get involved with.

KINKY

Colette is a 36-year-old music teacher. All her life she has led a pretty sheltered existence. There are times when she wishes she could break out and be a little more outgoing, but on the whole she is pretty happy with her lot.

An only child, she lives with her ageing mother in a large house in the middle of the city. She is a handsome-looking woman with a voluptuous figure that she hides under very conservative clothes. She looks very Home Counties.

Recently she met a man in a most unusual way when her umbrella got caught in his basket while they were shopping at Tesco. It made them both laugh, especially when he said, 'We must stop meeting like this.' To her surprise she countered with, 'How original.'

Over a coffee in the huge shopping complex, they laughed and joked and agreed to meet up again. Three dates later and now Ralph thinks they should become more intimate. But Colette is not so sure.

THE DREAM
I am at a dungeon party where everybody is dressed in outrageous leather and rubber outfits. I am wearing my normal clothes and feel very conspicuous. In the corner a man is down on all fours and a woman with impossibly high black patent stilettos has one foot on his back. Another man is wearing a tiny rubber posing pouch and what looks like a gas mask.

I cannot move; I am rooted to the floor in horrified fascination. A woman walks past me and she is dressed in a rubber outfit that looks like the kind of thing that the singer Madonna would wear. It has huge cones where her breasts are and her navel is pierced with a chain running from a ring up to the tips of the cones.

A man approaches me and says, 'Here, put these on — you'll need them.' As if in a trance I take off my clothes, letting them fall in a heap on the ground.

I step into the rubber boots and slip on the rubber coat he gives me, rushing to tie the belt as he leads me to a door. He opens it and I step through. Suddenly everything is bright and airy and I am standing in front of a small pond. 'Feed the ducks,' he says as I realise I am wearing a rain mac and wellington boots.

ANALYSIS

This dream shows the contradictions that make all of our personalities up. Colette's prudish old-fashioned approach breaks through in a very sexy dream. What she can take from the dream is that it is all right to let yourself go and take precautions at the same time, whether that means emotionally or in terms of safe sex.

However, she should not feel pushed into doing anything that she doesn't feel comfortable with and she should tell Ralph how she feels. If he really is serious about her then he will respect her feelings.

KISS

Celeste is a 28-year-old legal secretary who has been going out with Mark for five years. All around her, friends are getting married and more recently she was at her best friend's wedding, and caught the bouquet. Later on at the wedding Mark whispered in her ear that he thought it was a good idea for them to get hitched too. Celeste laughed the idea off and Mark was offended, questioning her commitment to him after so many years.

But the truth is that their sex life doesn't set her alight and she can't help but feel that her love life should be more passionate. She does love him and he is the only man she feels really close to but she can't help feeling that marriage is so final.

THE DREAM

Mark and I are getting ready to go out to dinner at a friend's house. He is ready before I am and as usual I can't find anything to wear. I'm getting into a really bad mood and I throw my clothes around the room. 'Look at me, I'm a bloody blob,' I say. 'It's only since we started living together that I put on all this weight. I must have put on at least a stone, none of it in the right places. I'm really fed up!'

But Mark is jovial and says, 'That's because you are content.' 'Yes, like a big fat pig at the trough,' I shout back before slamming the bathroom door. For no real reason I start to sob. He stands outside the bathroom and says, 'I think you are beautiful, even if you are a pig.'

Indignant, I fling open the door and he stands there

with his arms open, saying, 'Come here.' We hug and he says, 'You are the most beautiful person in the world and I love you,' then he kisses me.

As he does so I feel a warmth flow through me and I feel happy and safe again. He picks me up and carries me into the bedroom where he lays me on top of the pile of discarded clothes then presses his body to mine. And all the time we are kissing like I have never kissed before.

ANALYSIS
Kissing in a dream is a good sign. It is particularly relevant for Celeste because in her situation the kiss represents lasting happiness. She says that everything else is right about her relationship with Mark apart from their sex life. Initial passion is always spent quickly in all relationships and what replaces it is a deeper love and understanding. That passion can be rekindled by making time for love-making in the same way you would make time for eating a meal. Celeste should try taking the initiative one evening by preparing a night of seduction.

KNICKERS

Antonia has a new boyfriend, a handsome Italian. She is smitten with him but the only problem is a major one – the fact that he is married. He has told Antonia that his relationship with his wife is essentially over and that they are living separate lives. However, it will be some time before they are able to divorce because of his young son.

She has a niggling thought that Paolo is not telling the whole truth yet she puts it out of her mind when it crops up. And anyway he is spending his first full weekend with her soon. His wife is going on a trip with their son to visit her mother.

THE DREAM

I am at the hotel where Paolo and I have arranged to meet for the weekend. It is a beautiful sumptuous place with an old-world charm. I have arrived earlier as we arranged and he was going to follow on later to arrive in time for dinner.

It gives me just enough time to relax and have a really long scented bath. I have brought tons of creams, perfumes and make-up so that when he arrives I will look like a million dollars.

The crowning glory, though, is a pure silk bra and knickers set. Hand-made by La Perla, they are ivory-coloured with deep rich lace. Stripping off to jump into the bath, I try them on. They look exquisite.

I put them back into their tissue box and place them back in the top drawer of the dressing table, squeezing myself in delight.

As I soak in the bath, the phone rings and, dripping in

soap suds, I race to answer it. It is Paolo, who says he is sorry but he has to stay at home because his son has fallen ill and his wife expects him to be there. He says he will try to come to the hotel tomorrow but he doesn't know if he can make it or not.

I sit down on the bed, tears streaming down my face and I hit the pillow, crying, 'Why? Why?'

Then, in a fit of fury and disappointment, I open the drawer where the sexy underwear is and pulling out the tissue, I discover that the underwear is now just a pair of greying knickers.

I feel very confused.

ANALYSIS

Antonia knows in her heart she is onto a loser here. If she sits down and really thinks about the relationship she will realise that Paolo is like a great many men: he wants to have his cake and eat it. She is doing herself a disservice by putting her life on hold like this. She deserves a great deal more.

She is trying to build up the perfect love scenario, but that is impossible because she is starting off on a very flawed basis. If Paolo and his wife really do live separate lives then why does he have to wait until she goes away before he can spend a whole weekend with her?

The change of the beautiful underwear into tatty knickers shows that she is trying to create something beautiful out of something that is tawdry and worthless.

LEATHER

Oliver is a 32-year-old commodities dealer. Born into a poor background, he has always been driven to succeed and to earn money. For him money equals freedom equals power. He has achieved a lot of freedom, a stylish flat and a sporty Mercedes.

At work he lives a pressurised day, always trying to be top dog in his field. The rewards are great but the expectations placed upon him are also great.

THE DREAM

There is a group of Hell's Angels hanging around outside a motel. They are scruffy and quite menacing-looking and as I pull into the forecourt driving a pick-up truck, I feel a little apprehensive.

Their bikes are incredible to look at and I feel myself staring in awe. The gang go into the diner attached to the motel, leaving a woman with dirty blonde hair behind. She is bending over one of the bikes — it's a Harley — and I find myself admiring her chassis, not the bike's.

She catches my eye and says, 'Want a ride?' in a really sexy, smoky voice. It is an opportunity of a lifetime and I am not going to miss it. I hop up behind her and her leather skirt, which was short already, rides up even higher. She squeals in delight as we round corners at breakneck speed. I feel exhilarated and alive.

She pulls off the road and into a secluded wooded area, where she parks the bike. Then she French kisses me, thrusting her tongue deep into my throat. I am instantly aroused and respond vigorously to her hands running over my body. Then I turn her around and leaning her over the seat of the bike, I see she has no knickers on and I take her from behind until I'm spent.

Then we get back on to the bike and the last thing I remember is driving back up the road.

ANALYSIS

Take a holiday — you need a break. The presence of a motorbike in a dream indicates a need to re-evaluate your life, decide what is important to you and work towards it. All work and no play can make Jack or Oliver a dull boy.

Perhaps a trip on the open roads is just the tonic. Wild women and rampant unattached sex is one of the more common male dreams. The presence of leather in a dream indicates hard work to achieve an aim. In Oliver's case the leather-clad biker girl is the reward.

LECHERY

Forty-year-old Nick is a bored junior executive who cannot see a way up the career ladder. His wife is no longer interested in sex as it seemed that any time they attempted it, she got pregnant almost immediately. He has three boisterous boys who are into every kind of sport imaginable. Sometimes he just feels like a meal ticket and he thinks that the only reason anybody would miss him is if they didn't have his salary.

His last child was born seven years ago and since then his sex life has been practically non-existent. Lately he has started to look at lots of pornographic magazines and movies. He finds that he spends part of his day fantasising about the men and women in his office, wondering if they have a decent sex life.

THE DREAM

I am in my office on a cold and windy day and I am day-dreaming again, wondering what the women in my office are wearing underneath their boring office clothes. As I sit there I hit on the great idea of how I can finally find out.

There is an open staircase in the building where my office is. It's one of those which have gaps between the steps and it spirals slightly so that if you are underneath you can see right up women's skirts. The only problem is it is difficult to get in under there because the bottom of the stairs stops almost opposite the gents' loos.

But I work out that if I am down there before anybody else and I pretend to be on my mobile phone then I can look up their skirts without anyone thinking I'm a pervert.

I am in position by the time that everybody starts to leave. One by one they walk down and I am treated to a succession of my work colleagues' underwear: Tights, stockings and suspenders, white panties, black, red. Surprise, surprise, even the bosses' secretary, who has been with the company for more years than I can care to remember, is there and she's wearing suspenders and stockings. I've got a real bird's-eye view and I'm really enjoying it. When I wake up I am disappointed that the dream has ended.

ANALYSIS

This dream sounds like a case of wish-fulfilment. People who are not having sex or who have it very infrequently often have a lot of dreams about sex. Given Nick's personal background and his fascination with sex magazines, his dream shows that it is a problem that is preying on his mind. In any relationship there will be times when either or both partners are not in the mood for lovemaking. In these situations a caring partner will not feel rejected or pressurise their partner.

But when sex is a no-go area in a partnership, then it is unfair on the rejected partner to be expected to be happy with the arrangement. Constant rejection is unhealthy for a person's self-esteem. Nick and his wife need to address the problem of sex. It could be that their marriage is failing in other areas which then affect the way they both feel about each other. It is a dead-end approach not to deal with the problem.

LESBIANISM

Georgina, 19, has just started work as a beauty technician at a very up-market health club. It's her first job in London and coming from the country, she finds it a little bit daunting. She was pleased when Rachel, a senior technician, took her under her wing and showed her the town. Georgina and 23-year-old Rachel soon became the best of buddies.

Rachel was a real Londoner, born and bred in Islington. She was everything that Georgina wanted to be, street-wise, sassy and sophisticated when it was necessary. She had left home when she was just 17 and shared a flat with two other girls not far from the health club. Georgina often stayed there, sleeping on a sofa after a hard night's pubbing and clubbing.

THE DREAM

Rachel and I are in her bedroom trying on my clothes as I unpack them and put them into the wardrobe. I have just moved in and I am really excited to be there. Rachel has bought a bottle of cheap sparkling wine to drink a toast to my arrival.

Pretty soon we are laughing and giggling because the alcohol has started to take effect. Most of my stuff looks too big on Rachel because she is very slim and reed-like, while I am more curvy with quite a large bust.

She leaves the room and comes back with a sparkly spaghetti-strap dress and tells me to try it on. 'It's a little too big in the bust area for me and just hangs there. You'd fill it out better,' she says.

I feel a little shy and struggle to put the dress on without taking off my bra. 'Don't be silly,' she says. 'We've all got the same.' And with that she spins me around and undoes the hooks at the back of my bra, then she helps me to take it off.

The dress, a vibrant red, does look sensational but I feel exposed and I cover my chest, saying, 'I don't know if I could go out like this.'

'Nonsense,' Rachel says, 'you should be proud of them.' And she puts her two hands around my breasts and cups them. Then she kisses me on the mouth. I feel faint but excited, then I pull away from her all embarrassed. Then I woke up.

ANALYSIS

Like dreams of homosexuality, dreams of lesbianism in straight people do not mean your sexuality is in question. It is perfectly evident that Rachel is someone Georgina looks up to and that she wishes to try to emulate her. Lesbian scenes in dreams simply show that you, the dreamer, wants to attain qualities that the object of your desire has got. A positive message that Georgina can take from the dream is that she too has qualities that others would like to have — a curvy bust for a start!

MASTURBATION

Mary is a nurse who has recently been moved to the casualty department of the hospital she works in. She has ambitions to be a sister and felt the move would sharpen her up so that she works faster and more decisively.

What she didn't expect was the added difficulties of not having enough space for the patients to stay or the level of violence that is often directed at staff by distressed relatives or drunken yobs. She has also had to work overtime because of staff shortages. She feels there's not enough time to do anything. She had her dream after a particularly gruelling night shift.

THE DREAM
I am in a mirrored bathroom and in the middle there is a huge bath that is full of bubbles. The scent is delicious and reeks of luxury. It is the most inviting bath I've ever seen and I climb into it, revelling in its cosy warmth.

The room is illuminated by candlelight and I just sit and relax for ages. I lazily pick up the rose-scented soap and rub it over my shoulders and breasts. The frothy, creamy bubbles cover my nipples, which are beginning to harden.

I run my hands down my body, over my stomach and between my legs. There I explore the secret parts of me and tease and tweak my clitoris in a languid way. Arching my back, I rise out of the water and see my reflection in the mirrors and my fingers exploring my vagina.

As I submerge my body again, I can feel the orgasm building up until it sends waves of shudders through my body. My energy spent, I slump down into the bubbles and feel totally relaxed and at ease.

ANALYSIS

Masturbation in a dream is indicative of a need for the dreamer to relax and spend time on themselves. Mary feels the tension of her work and she is strung out. The message she can take from this dream is that she should make sure that she gets time to herself, even if it means just sitting on the sofa with a box of chocolates and a purring cat as she listens to gentle music.

MILE-HIGH CLUB

Sam, 26, has been seeing a woman who is intelligent, witty and beautiful. It seems as if she has got it all and that he is a very lucky man. But he finds her a little daunting. She is very outgoing and is always making new friends, whereas he is quite reserved and would rather watch from the sidelines than jump in. Paula is usually the life and soul of the party and often drags Sam up to dance, but he feels self-conscious.

THE DREAM

Paula and I are at the airport on our way to Barbados for a holiday. We both have tans even though we haven't even left Britain. I'm feeling quite excited at the prospect of two weeks in the sun and lots of ice-cold drinks.

We check in and after a while we board the plane. As soon as the plane takes off, I arrange for some champagne to be brought and we toast our holiday. She's giggly and loving, kissing me on the ear as she leans across me to look out of the window.

Then she says, 'Let's join the Mile-High Club.' At first I didn't know what she meant but when she explained it I felt a bit panicky. Then she told me I was an old fuddy-duddy and challenged me to break out. The champagne was beginning to take effect so I said yes, but later.

The dream skipped to a few hours later when everybody was busy watching a movie. Paula went down to the loo and after a few seconds I joined her, knocking on the door three times like she told me.

As soon as I walked in she grabbed me and kissed me.

It was tiny in there and the only way we could do it was by me sitting down on the seat and her straddling me. She had bare legs and was wearing strappy white sandals. Her top was open and she was highly excited.

The next thing I remember is sitting back in my seat as the air hostess served drinks and seeing Paula return. As she sat down she put a pair of knickers in my lap and I nearly dropped my coffee.

ANALYSIS

Travelling by plane and indeed joining the Mile-High Club is indicative of Sam's efforts to shed his inhibitions. He is unsure about his commitment to Paula because he finds her hot to handle. Rather than let the relationship just drag along with him feeling uncomfortable, he should talk to her and explain that he must be allowed the space to be himself and not conform to what she wants every time. He could also think about relaxing a little more so that they meet on common ground.

MOTHER-IN-LAW

Gabriel recently lost his job and after a long battle to keep up the mortgage on the house he and his wife, Marlene, bought, they had to sell up. The debts were beginning to be crippling. Tragically, they had been married only six months and had worked hard to build a home.

Consequently the young couple had to move in with Marlene's mother, who lives by herself not far from where their own home was. Marlene's father died when she was 18 and since then her mother had come to depend on her only child for everything, but mainly for company.

Needless to say, Marlene's mother resented their relationship and it took years before there was an easy peace between her and Gabriel. Now he is forced to spend his days with her as he job-hunts. She is very disapproving of him and when her daughter returns home she makes a big fuss of her, telling her she shouldn't have to work so hard.

Gabriel had the following dream.

THE DREAM

My wife and I are in bed in her old bedroom. As we snuggle down she kisses me and tells me she loves me. She is naked but I am wearing pyjamas because I feel I should cover up. She coaxes me to take them off and starts kissing me as she undoes each button until she gets to my navel. She continues on as she takes off the bottoms of the set.

Paula has a beautiful curvy body and as she sits across my legs I marvel at the sight of her. The duvet tumbles to the ground as I pull her under me and begin kissing her.

As I enter her I feel so much love for her. Our passions mount as our lovemaking becomes more energetic. Suddenly the door opens as I am in mid-stroke and her mother walks in, dragging a vacuum cleaner with her.

'It's only me,' she says. 'You two carry on.' I am dumb-struck, especially when Paula says, 'Thanks for doing that, Mum,' as the machine kicks into life.

ANALYSIS

Mothers-in-law always get a bad press. To dream of one means that you are facing a difficult situation that will need to be handled with great diplomacy.

Sam feels invaded as though she comes between him and Paula. Although the couple are staying at her house she really ought to give them the breathing space that they need.

The best way this situation can be handled is for Paula to talk to her mother and try to arrange a satisfactory arrangement for all concerned. That way they can all make the best of a bad lot until their fortunes change for the better.

NATURISM

Howard is a hard-nosed sales manager who is ambitious and hard-working. He hasn't got any real friends at work and until now he can't say it has ever really bothered him that much. Recently, however, he was in a cubicle in the men's toilets when he overheard a conversation being held about him.

'He's a tough bastard,' said one of his sales team.

'Operates like a lone wolf,' agreed the other. 'I wonder what he's like out of work?' To which the second man replied, 'It's probably best we don't find out.'

THE DREAM

I'm on holiday playing frisbee with my dog. He's a huge golden Labrador and as I throw it, he races along and catches it before bringing it back to me. Then a woman with a mongrel walks past and he is distracted from the game. He runs after the other dog and I have to get my wife to hold on to him while I retrieve the frisbee.

As I look for it in the clump of grass, I notice that there is a sign which announces the start of the nudist beach. Curious, I throw the frisbee so that it goes past the sign and I have to follow. It gives me the opportunity to take a quick peek.

There aren't many people on the beach, but those that are there aren't wearing any clothes and seem to act perfectly normally.

I go back and tell my wife and she suggests we try it. 'It'll be the first time I ever get an all-over tan, she says.' I refuse – but the next day while she's having beauty treatment I go back to the nudist beach. While I'm stand-ing there a couple see me as they go on to that section.

'Try it, it's very liberating,' says the woman as she strips off her swimsuit. Eventually I do. At first I felt a bit silly, afraid I'd get an erection but then I felt so free letting it all hang loose.

ANALYSIS

Going naked in a dream can reveal two things. Unwanted nudity in a dream can be distressing. But in Howard's case it can be liberating. He would dearly love to drop his façade at work, yet feels he cannot because his persona is carved in stone as far as the staff are concerned. This dream shows a desire to reveal the true self for a change.

NECROPHILIA

Hugh has been involved in an on-off relationship for some time now with his girlfriend, Ann-Marie. It is a stormy relationship at the best of times, their two strong personalities clashing badly all the time. Yet they can't stay away from each other for long. The most recent separation has been the longest they have ever gone without relenting and calling each other.

He is torn between his feelings for her and the realisation that they do not seem to be suited.

THE DREAM

I am in a mortuary, being led through a set of double doors. They close quietly behind me and I am alone with a body laid out on a cold marble slab. It is Ann-Marie and sobbing, I walk to her side. She looks beautiful, as though she is just sleeping, with her black hair fanned out behind her head.

I stand staring at her for ages then I bend down and kiss her. She seems warm and I feel she is alive and responding to me. I put my hand on her waist and feel she is naked beneath the sheet.

'It's the last time I'll ever see or feel you,' I say to her. As I caress her still body I feel a stirring in my loins. The next thing I am on top of her, my trousers round my ankles as I prepare to make love to her. At that moment a mortuary attendant walks in and catches me. He looks horrified and it hits me like a thunderbolt what I was doing. I slump to the ground devastated and sobbing. When I wake up I am crying.

ANALYSIS

Hugh must realise that his relationship with Ann-Marie is dead. In the dream he attempts to make love to a lifeless corpse. The symbolism of the corpse is that what he had with Ann-Marie earlier on in their relationship is now dead. Difficult as that may be to accept he must move on and resist the temptation to contact her again.

NUDITY

Ollie is a sharp, dapper 23-year-old advertising sales rep on a busy daily newspaper, who works long hours, enjoys playing hard with the boys in the bar and revels in his off-duty status as a toyboy. He had lived with ad agency executive Barbara, who is ten years his senior, for only two months before this dream.

Privately Ollie is far more shy than his work mates could ever imagine and almost painfully conscious that Barbara always takes the lead during sex. She is a mature, confident woman, aware of and perfectly at ease with her own sexuality and physical needs.

Ollie, however, longs to assert his manhood as the dominant partner, yet is afraid he will be perceived as clumsy, ungainly or even worse, a failure in bed. The couple enjoy a comfortable lifestyle but Ollie is beset by nagging doubts about their long-term future.

THE DREAM

I'm dressed in a designer suit, looking the business, as I knock on the front door. Someone opens it and there is a blast of party noise, loud music and laughter. As I walk in nobody pays any attention to me. It is a beautiful house, very up-market and sophisticated.

Then I see Barbara standing at the end of the bar, looking stunning in a long, black evening dress. She catches my eyes, smiles and then it's as if everything is in slow motion. I realise I have got a drink in my hand and I can sense the glass is at an angle and I'm spilling its contents.

Before I look down I notice that Barbara is not smiling

at me, she is laughing. As I look around everyone at the party is laughing at me. Feeling a terrible sense of dread, I look down and realise that I am naked. The laughter seems to get louder and I can feel myself heat up. Shame and humiliation overwhelm me and I wake up.

ANALYSIS

Nudity is a common dream symbol which reflects the dreamer's feelings of deep anxiety or vulnerability. Although on the surface Ollie seems confident, it is mainly an act. He feels stripped of confidence, laid bare before his all-knowing partner.

He must confide his feeling of inferiority to Barbara, who, if she really loves him, will help create a more relaxed atmosphere where they are equal as lovers despite the age difference.

ORAL SEX

Sian got a little drunk on New Year's Eve and had unprotected sex with a friend of a friend. She didn't even ask him his surname and they certainly didn't have any intention of seeing each other again.

Since then she has felt terribly guilty about it and spent a month worrying that she might have been pregnant. But thankfully she was not. Even then she can't seem to shake off the guilt she feels.

THE DREAM

I am in a kind of fairground booth, like the kind that Gypsy Rose Lee the fortune-teller would have. It's all stripy in blue and white. Outside there are signs telling people to come into the tent and try my wonderful skills.

A man comes in through the door, takes down his trousers and presents me with his erect member. I give him oral sex and he leaves after zipping up. Straight away another man comes in and does the same thing and I give him oral sex until he empties himself in my mouth.

This goes on for ages with what seems like dozens of men taking advantage of my oral service. I wake up just as another man walks through the curtained door.

I felt really disgusted with myself because I've never even had oral sex. What can it mean?

ANALYSIS

In dreams parts of the body often do not represent exactly what they seem to be. More often than not the mouth,when it is the focus of a dream, is a symbol for the vagina. Sian's preoccupation with her rampant one-night stand is the root of this dream. What she forgot to do was to check that she had not picked up any venereal diseases.

It may be that she does not want to face that fact and therefore she is putting it to the back of her mind. However, the niggling thought will be there until she gets the all-clear on her health.

ORGASM

Guy is a 17-year-old student who has only just realised there are girls out there. He has always concentrated on his studies rather than romance so he is lagging behind his mates when it comes to experience. In fact he is a virgin and finds it excruciatingly embarrassing when they talk about their first time or the latest girlfriend and how far she is prepared to go.

He has tried to cover up his lack of experience but his friends are not fooled. He feels like his virginity is a huge cross to bear and is keen to get rid of it.

THE DREAM

I am in my bedroom and the door opens. A really gorgeous woman walks in — she looks like Cindy Crawford. She is wearing one of those silky negligées and her legs are tanned and smooth. She climbs into the bed with me and kisses me with her red lips.

I'm not quite sure what to do and I am clumsy and fumbling. She guides my hand to the thin strap of her negligée and indicates for me to slip it down over her arms.

She has beautiful breasts, really pert, and they are so soft to touch. I am surprised by their softness. She wiggles out of the silky garment and stands beside my bed naked. I'm running my hands over her body, really enjoying myself. I am ready for action, but I'm not really sure what I should do. I feel a bit stupid.

But she takes the initiative and lies down on the bed, then pulls me on top of her. It feels really awkward at first but she guides me inside her. Then I let myself go and move with the rhythms of her body. It seemed like only seconds before I orgasmed. When I woke up I was lying on my front making the same movements on the bed as though I was really making love.

ANALYSIS
What Guy had was essentially a wet dream. People who dream of orgasms normally do not enjoy an active sex life, and have a need to release tension. This is a wish-fulfilment dream — the dream many male fans of women like Cindy Crawford would like to experience. The fact is that when the right girl comes along and the time feels right, then Guy's first experience of sex will be a positive one and he should not think of his virginity merely as unwanted baggage to be dumped.

ORGY

Patricia, who is 15, recently started to hang out with a girl she met at the school disco. Sharon is in another class but Patricia had often seen her in the corridor and thought that she looked a little bit wild but great fun.

When Patricia spoke to her in the toilets at the disco she was surprised at how pleasant she actually was. Now Sharon has invited her to go away for a weekend at a friend's parents' house to celebrate one of the gang's birthday. She is keen to go but feels a little bit apprehensive as she doesn't know any of the others.

THE DREAM
I am in a strange house and there are masses of people all over the place. I go upstairs to the bathroom. There are three doors and because I don't know which one leads where, I open up the nearest one. It's really dark and I can hear moaning.

I switch the light on, and a chorus of voices shout, 'Switch it off!' I do so but I have had just enough time to see that the room is not a bathroom, but a bedroom. Sprawled across the bed are at least six naked bodies. As my eyes adjust to the light again I can see that they are having sex. It's like an orgy. There are couples doing all sorts of things and one girl is being fondled by two men at the same time.

'Come on in,' a voice from the gloom says and a girl gets up from the bed and takes my hand. I pull away from her and shake my head. I really don't want to go into the room. I close the door and open up the one to the bathroom.

Then I wake up really surprised at such a dream, and also feeling a little embarrassed.

ANALYSIS

This is a warning from Patricia's subconscious in response to her real-life hesitancy about going to stay with a crowd of strangers. The dream indicates that she needs to be careful about the company she keeps. She clearly felt that the gang would be rather wild, as she thought Sharon was at first, and that they might get up to things she would not be comfortable with.

There is no need for her not to be friends with Sharon but perhaps she ought to get to know her a little better before taking the plunge by going away with her and a group of strangers.

PORNOGRAPHY

Julia, 40, has been married to her childhood sweetheart for 15 years and she is bored. Their two children are relatively independent and her husband has a daily routine from which he never deviates. She feels that there has to be more to life, yet when she tries to discuss it with her husband he tells her she is imagining problems and that he is quite content with the way things are.

She knows it is fanciful thinking, but she wishes she could turn the clock back to a time when everything seemed more exciting.

THE DREAM

I am in a huge studio with lots of lights and cameras and those big white boards they use. There is a photographer and somebody helping him with the cameras. The music is loud and heavy but very uplifting. I am standing with a glass of champagne while they mess around with the equipment. I am wearing a very glamorous lace and satin side-split dress.

'All right darlin', let's go,' says the photographer. I walk over to one of those huge cane chairs that you used to see in houses in the seventies. I sit down and he starts to take pictures of me, issuing instructions all the time: 'lean forward', 'hold your arms together', 'more bust', 'more leg'.

I go through a whole series of poses until I am stripped off down to my underwear. The photographer comes over and shows me some Polaroids he has done, praising me and telling me that I am a stunner. I feel very pleased and very special that anyone would want to photograph me.

Then we start shooting again and this time I am taking off all my clothes and really playing up to the camera, pouting and posing. I feel really happy.

ANALYSIS

Poor Julia. She and countless other women experience indifference at a certain point in their marriages. This dream reflects her unhappiness at the lack of attention from her husband and indeed her two children. She feels like a spent penny. Being photographed in this way indicates that she craves stimulation and would love to be desired and adored. The problem with many marriages like Julia's is that there comes a time when the couple stop really communicating with each other. Instead they just assume that the other knows how they feel and think. But we all change and the lesson she can learn from this dream is that she should try to introduce some excitement into the relationship. In that way she might coax her husband out of a rigid pattern of life which he too probably finds boring but which he doesn't know how to change. He may well then see her once again as a flesh-and-blood person, deserving of the attention he has deprived her of for so long.

PROMISCUITY

For years Toby had always hidden his true sexuality. Instead he buried himself in his studies at first and later on his work as an architect. Whenever his family asked him why he never seemed to have a steady relationship, he would dismiss it by saying he was too career-minded.

The truth was that Toby was not interested in women; he was gay. He didn't tell his family because he thought they couldn't take the truth, they would be horrified. His parents had always had stereotyped attitudes towards families and sex.

It wasn't until he moved to London to take up a new position with a large progressive firm that he began to live more openly. Freed from the shackles of convention, he was like a child let loose in a sweet shop. He wanted to try everything and everyone.

THE DREAM

I am in a prison — like one of those huge American ones that you see in films. There are tiers of cells accessed by metal walkways. I am being brought in wearing handcuffs and I go through a series of gates accompanied by prison officers who are grim-faced.

As I walk past the streams of prisoners some of them sneer at me and others ignore me. There are all nationalities and colours here. I feel a little apprehensive, especially when one of the guards start to laugh when another asks who I'm sharing my cell with.

I am led, carrying a bunch of blankets up the stairs past a long line of closed cell doors. 'Nice ass,' is a comment I hear over and over again and several wolf-whistle as I pass.

In my cell I am astonished at how small it is and before I even go in I feel claustrophobic. There is a huge black guy on the bottom bunk. As I walk in he glares at me. The door is slammed shut and I turn around to look through the bars.

'Welcome to paradise,' the guy says and I feel his hand on my waist. Down below another batch of prisoners are being led into the main area. I feel trapped and wake up with a really anxious feeling.

ANALYSIS

This is a dream forewarning Toby of the dangers of his liberated behaviour. He is indeed like a child in a sweet shop, and a child allowed to run riot and eat whatever he or she likes will inevitably get sick. Toby may be feeling more liberated than he has ever felt in his life, but he must treat that liberty with caution.

He has gone from celibacy to promiscuity and that can spell danger. Dreaming of being in prison is warning him to be careful before his behaviour lands him in trouble. Promiscuity can lead to infectious diseases, so he must either protect himself properly or curb his activities.

PROSTITUTION

Martine has been going out with Ernest, a Dutchman, for six months. She is a very attractive woman, with blonde hair and blue eyes. She has always relied on her physical attributes rather than her brains and hard work to see her through life.

So it is no surprise that Ernest, who spends a lot of time travelling in his work, tends to treat her as a bimbo when he is in town. He is an arrogant man who is very clever when it comes to business, but when it comes to women he goes for a good arm decoration. Martine fits the bill, but when she tries to voice an opinion, he dismisses her.

However, she is seduced by the glitzy lifestyle he can afford to give her: expensive restaurants, beautiful presents and a chauffeur-driven Jaguar.

THE DREAM
It's a dark and dingy street; it's cold and there is a feeling of desperation about the place. I am walking along with another woman who is chewing gum and talking really fast. She is dressed in a really short skirt and high, black-patent stilettos. Her blouse is frilly and you can see her bra through it.

I am wearing a shiny red satin skirt and really high thigh boots. They are a little uncomfortable to walk in and I have a slight limp.

The woman and I agree to stand near each other, and it is then that I realise I am a prostitute. Within a very short space of time the woman climbs into a car with a client.

I am by myself when I see a Jaguar turn into the road;

it crawls along the kerb past the other women — there seem to be about half a dozen of them there. It slows down beside me and a window winds down. A face appears from the dark interior and says, 'Are you doing business?'

'Of course,' I reply and move towards the door. But just as I've got my hand on the handle the voice says, 'I've changed my mind. Driver, that looks like a better deal over there.'

I look up and there is a younger-looking version of me touting for business. As the car pulls away, I see the contours of the man's face and it's Ernest.

ANALYSIS

It's obvious that Martine is selling herself. Until now it was something that she could handle, but Ernest's attitude towards her makes her feel devalued as a person. She needs either to get out of this relationship or, if she truly has any feeling for the man, stand her ground and see what happens. The ball is in her court now and she has to decide if she wants to kick it.

QUICKIE SEX

Michael is a truck driver who is often away from home as he drives in Europe quite a lot. He has been married to Tricia for four years and loves her dearly. He knows that when he is away she is not going to play around, and will always be faithful to him.

He finds that the conversation among his fellow truck drivers often turns to sex. They are full of stories about all the women they pick up on their travels and their exploits in their trucks' sleeping compartments.

Michael would never be unfaithful to Tricia, but he can't help but be intrigued by the sexual experience some of these women seem to have and he wishes that his demure little wife wasn't so demure sometimes. She is strictly missionary position and anything else would not be tolerated.

THE DREAM

It's a dark night and I am in my cabin parked outside a roadside café. I have the radio on and I am reading a magazine by the light of a lamp above my head. I don't feel very sleepy.

Suddenly I hear the sounds of footsteps crunching on the gravel outside my truck. I hold my breath and I feel anxious. You never know who is going to turn up as you sleep by the roadside. Reaching under my pillow I pull out the axe-handle I keep in case of emergency.

Someone climbs on to my truck and tries the handle of the door. It's locked.

I'm angry now and keyed up, so I climb into the front

and fling the door on the other side open, jump down and with the axe-handle raised I run around the other side of the truck.

A woman giggles; she is leaning against the body of the truck, in semi-darkness. Still nervous, I demand to know what she wants.

'You,' she says, walking towards me.

It's Tricia and she is dressed like a real tart with a skirt right up her backside. I am standing there in just my boxer shorts and before I can say anything she leans forward and pulls them down, then says, 'Do it to me.'

I need no more encouragement and I pull her on to me while still standing and enter her without even taking off her clothes — she's not wearing any knickers anyway.

I orgasm very quickly and slump back against the cabin step. She stands up, straightens her skirt and smiling, walks away.

ANALYSIS

There is a strong tinge of wish-fulfilment in this dream. Sex is important in a relationship and even more so when you are spending time apart. There is always temptation out there for everyone, but when you are on the road it's even greater as loneliness sets in and the need to be close to someone is strong.

Michael loves his wife but wishes she had a streak of excitement in her. However, they can work on it together and it is best to get started now rather than later. He could always begin by buying her some raunchy under-wear and encouraging her to express herself.

RAPE

Karen works as a secretary in a small office owned by a window glazing firm. There is also another secretary there, Sue. Between them they handle all the work generated by the sales reps and by the sales manager, Roger.

Roger is a bit two-faced and he tries to play the two girls off each other, favouring one of them one day and ignoring the other. They each have their turn at being the favourite. It really annoys Karen as she feels that kind of behaviour is detrimental to her career prospects. But she knows that if she left, knowing Roger as she does, he would not give her a good reference. She feels torn and does not look forward to work now.

THE DREAM

I need to go to the toilet and I tell Roger. He smiles and says, 'You go right ahead.' He is dressed in a greeny-grey suit, white shirt and a tie that has a lot of red in it.

I walk into the ladies' and to my surprise he is there, sitting on the ground with just a shirt and Y-fronts on. He looks a little drunk.

Then Sue comes in. He doesn't say it but I know he wants us to have sex with him. I feel very trapped and angry, but I daren't say anything.

I go to use the loo and by this stage he is standing above me — for some reason the loo is down a few steps. As I prepare to use it, he is leaning at the top looking at me. I feel very invaded but still I say nothing.

I don't use the loo and instead walk to go out of the ladies'. Sue has gone out already.

As I go to leave he grabs me by the hand and pushes me to the ground. The floor is cold, but I don't fight back. Then he spreads my legs and enters me, as I lie there like a dummy. When he is finished he leans back against the wall and holding his privates, says, 'What d'ya think of these then — aren't they beauts?'

I stand up, look at him and then walk over to him and give him a powerful kick in his 'beauts'. I feel really good and wake up laughing.

ANALYSIS

Dreams of rape are not sexual dreams, just like rape is usually nothing to do with sex in real life. Rapists are turned on by the power they wield over their victims. In Karen's dream she gets raped, but she fights back. She is being 'screwed' by Roger in her working life and she does nothing about it. Her dream's message is, 'Do something about it!' She must break the powerful hold he has over her.

ROMANCE

Molly has been living with Jed for a year and a half. They bought their flat together and she feels that he is not facing the responsibility of jointly owning a home like he should. Initially it was Molly who did all the decorating and put aside money to buy things like a fridge-freezer and the chairs they needed to furnish the place.

Their home is functional now but she's not happy with the way it looks. In fact she is wondering if she has made a mistake by committing herself to Jed. It is not only the furniture that annoys her: He also expects her to do all the housework and it is only after a stand-up argument that he will reluctantly wash and dry the dishes. He puts everything on the back burner and is a real 'tomorrow man'.

THE DREAM

I have a chance encounter with an ex-boyfriend as I am walking through a hotel lobby. I work there and he is a guest. We are both really happy to see each other and give each other huge hugs. I am just finishing work and Jim is here on a course. We go into the bar to have a drink and he, always the romantic, orders a bottle of champagne.

He raises a toast to me and says, 'The years have been good to you.' We chat for ages and it's getting late. I tell him I really must go, but I don't want to. He asks me to stay for dinner and I relent. We are seated in the dining room, which has beautiful starched linen tablecloths. All around us there are couples who are sitting in the light of the small candles in the middle of the tables.

Jim orders the food: oysters. When they come he feeds

me one from the shell and pays undivided attention to everything I say. Then we dance to a waltz in the really old-fashioned way and he kisses my hand, saying, 'We should never have parted.' I feel really guilty about Jed as I really don't want to leave Jim.

I am looking at Jim in my dream and just thinking about how comfortable I feel with him and how I wish things could be like the early days. But I know that they won't and that you can never go back. I tell him I have to go and he looks disappointed, but he walks me to the front of the hotel and kisses me gently on the mouth before handing me a red rose. 'I'll always love you, Molly,' he says. I watch him walk away and feel a terrible sense of sadness and loss.

ANALYSIS

When a woman dreams of an old boyfriend, it does not necessarily mean that she wants to turn back the clock for real. Molly obviously split up because there was something wrong with her relationship in the beginning. However, it is more probable that she is isolating the qualities that she identified as good in her ex-boyfriend.

There are obviously qualities in Jim that she wishes Jed had, but they are two separate people and she must either accept that or move on.

Jed sounds selfish and immature. Every time she tries to discuss anything it ends in a slanging match. Jim, on the other hand, listens to her every word. Molly should try writing down with complete honesty how she feels. Alternatively, she could take off for a holiday, and perhaps then Jed will realise what he has got in her. It will also give her a chance to think clearly about what she wants in life.

RUDE LANGUAGE

Jason's girlfriend, Teresa, is driving him crazy. She is deeply insecure about their relationship no matter how hard he tries to reassure her. They live together and she is always saying he doesn't care about her.

Whenever she is going through one of her traumas, she hates everything, including herself. She is constantly asking him if she is fat. If he says no, she asks the question a different way. No matter what the answer is she is still not happy. It confuses him that she won't believe him and he has got to the stage where he is very careful about the answers he gives. Nowadays, more often than not he refuses even to comment, saying he has no opinion.

THE DREAM
I am rolling around in bed with a woman who I presume is my girlfriend. We are having a really rampant sex session and trying all different positions. It's great fun. Then she pushes me off gently and tells me to seduce her. She lies back on the pillow and using really rude language instructs me on what she wants.

I am slightly shocked but find the naughty language a turn-on. At her instruction I do what she says, starting at her breasts, moving on to her stomach and then down to her pubic area. She wants me to give her oral sex and all the time she is instructing me in what to do.

But my performance is not very good and she is getting a little irate; as I am down there she is still issuing instructions. I tell her I don't understand and she glares at me and starts talking again but I don't understand a word, as she is speaking a foreign language at a very fast speed. I just look at her really puzzled.

ANALYSIS

Communication is a problem with this couple, as is Teresa's lack of confidence. Jason is rightly confused by what she is saying because although they talk, she twists everything he says and that makes him unhappy. He feels as though nothing will please her. He is right about that, because unless she accepts herself, he is wasting his time. He should talk seriously about the problem and let her know that he is trying hard to please her, but she must be made to realise the effect of her behaviour on him and their relationship.

SADISM

Cynthia has been working on building sites for only three months. She is an electrician and being one of few women in the business, she is prone to a lot of sexual harassment and joking. She hates the early mornings, the wet days, the hard toil. But more than any of those things she hates the foreman, Bill.

A burly hulk of a man, Bill prides himself on being hard and he is always out to prove it. He doesn't like Cynthia as he thinks she should be at home having babies. At every opportunity he tries to ridicule her in front of the lads. Knowing that Cynthia hates heights, he delights in sending her up the scaffolding on silly errands.

THE DREAM

I have got Bill tied to the concrete-mixer, his trousers are around his ankles and I am whipping him with some electric cable. He is begging for mercy but I won't pay attention to his pleas.

I am dressed in a dominatrix outfit and I feel really powerful and dominant. After untying him I lead him up the stairs to the top floor by a collar I have put around his neck. If he doesn't walk fast enough then he starts to choke.

When I get him upstairs, I make him sit on the cold concrete floor. He is swearing at me, calling me a bitch. I tell him he's right about that. Then I get the jump leads I left attached to the car battery and holding one lead in each hand I click them like a crab clicking its claws as I walk across the empty, dusty office space.

He's whimpering now and I attach one of the leads to his manhood and the other to his ear, then very deliberately I walk back to the battery and toy with the switch. He is screaming now and is not very brave. Then I flick the switch and he tenses up, but nothing happens. I was only teasing. I walk over to him and say, 'Now Bill, I am very angry with you, but I will let you off just this once. Do you promise to behave in future?'

As he is nodding and thanking me for not doing anything I wake up. I am smiling at the dream, but I'd never dream of doing anything like that in real life.

ANALYSIS

Cynthia is too timid. If she wants to work in a man's world, especially the building trade, she has to get tough or, as she has already found out, she will continue to get walked over. Dreams involving sadism do not mean that there is a really dangerous part of the dreamer that would delight in torturing people. What this dream is saying to Cynthia is simply that she must not behave in such a timid fashion, but must stand up for herself.

SEX SLAVE

Jenny has been married for 25 years to Maurice. They are both in their early fifties. Maurice recently suffered a stroke which left him confined to a wheelchair. The couple have two children, both studying for exams. This has meant that the burden of looking after their father and them has fallen solely on Jenny, who feels drained emotionally and physically. Maurice is unable to even help share simple decision-making because he has sunk into a deep depression over his disability. Previously he was a dynamic self-employed wine shipper, but his company had to be sold.

Jenny had the following dream.

THE DREAM

I am in an exotic, temple-like building, in a room which is draped in fine, gauzy silk curtains. Scattered on the floor are huge, squashy embroidered cushions on which young women lounge. They are all clad only in Arabian Nights-style clothing, all veils, bare midriffs and jewellery. A few are eating fresh fruit from ornate bowls while others paint their nails different shades of red.

At the door, two huge men stand guard, their arms folded. The door flies open and an important-looking man enters. He points towards me, crooking his finger as if beckoning me to follow. I rise and walk obediently behind him as he turns back towards the door. We reach a hallway, walk through another huge, ornate door and there, in the middle of the room, is a giant bed. A naked man lies sprawling in the middle, paying no attention whatsoever to our entrance. Without my even noticing, the man I followed into the room has vanished.

Two women come into the room carrying bowls of water and scented oil. I am stripped down and washed then the oil is massaged into my body as I stand there. My nipples are tweaked so that they stand erect. I am ready and presented to the man on the bed. 'Ah, slave,' he says as I stand by the side of the bed. 'Come here and take me in your mouth.' I perform oral sex on him and he is quickly satisfied. He makes me lie on the bed beside him until he is erect again.

He clambers off the bed and tells me to lie face down, then, with his ready manhood, he penetrates me deeply and takes me doggy-fashion until he is satisfied. At this point I awake.

ANALYSIS

Jenny has had to shoulder all responsibility and it is weighing heavily on her now. A dream of this nature where the dreamer is a slave, of any kind, reflects the desire to throw off the mantle of responsibility.

She is exhausted and wants a let-up of the demands on her, even if it is just for a while. This is a warning dream: Jenny needs to take care of her own needs before she burns out from looking after others.

STRANGER

Louise is a PA in a PR firm. She knows that she could be something more than she is but she is not confident enough to handle the media. Some of that stems from her appearance, for she is overweight and feels self-conscious about it. But whenever her boss is about to do a new launch or organise a photo-call, she is always full of ideas, most of which are taken on board.

Now her boss wants her to concentrate more on the PR aspect of her work as she thinks she has valuable talents in that direction.

THE DREAM

I am travelling home on a train; it is early in the evening but the rush hour has finished so that the carriage is pretty empty. There is only another woman and a man in the carriage.

I am sitting opposite the man and the woman is to my left in another seat. She gets out about four stops from where I live. I am reading a Michael Crichton novel, *Disclosure*, when suddenly the train shudders to a halt.

The book goes flying and so do I, right into the lap of the man in front of me. I am really embarrassed. But he picks up the book and hands it back to me. 'Good book,' he says. 'Sexual harassment of a man, it's hard to believe. I think the guy is lucky — I've never been sexually harassed in my life.'

A mischievous idea comes into my mind and cheekily I say, 'What? A good-looking man like you? I could soon change that.'

155

'Try me,' he replied. I put my hand on his knee and moved it up his leg. He just sat there not moving, but had a big smile on his face. He was quite cute. Then I moved over to sit beside him and undid two of his shirt buttons.

I could see he was responding by the bulge in his trousers, so I deftly unzipped him, then getting him to move in the seat so that I could straddle him, I had sex with him. He still had all his clothes on. He responded with urgent thrusts and we both orgasmed together.

Almost immediately the train started to move again and I stood up while he tidied himself. I just managed to pull myself together again before we entered the next station — my stop. I didn't say a thing to him, just walked off the train, smiled and closed the door.

ANALYSIS

This dream was very risqué. The message that Louise can draw from it is that inside all of us there is a stranger waiting to be befriended. Louise saw a different aspect of herself that she is not yet familiar with. We all have abilities and resources that we do not tap into, and Louise should try the offer of becoming a full-time PR. Once she gets more experience, her confidence will grow. She is merely using her being overweight as an excuse to hide behind.

TELEPHONE SEX

Gina recently joined a dating agency because she has found it almost impossible to meet a partner since she works long hours in her job. She is a very ambitious person and her private life tends to suffer the consequences.

She is not a shrinking violet by any means — just a very practical person. Meeting people like this does have its down-side and Gina is aware of the dangers of meeting strangers in this fashion. Since she joined she has had several phone calls but has not yet committed herself to meeting anyone.

No one else knows that Gina has joined the agency, not even her best friend, as she feels slightly embarrassed about having done so.

THE DREAM
As I walk past a telephone box, the phone inside begins to ring. It startles me at first. There is no one waiting to answer it. At first I ignore it and continue on my way, but the incessant ringing makes me wonder who it is.

Curiosity gets the better of me and I turn back, open the door and pick up the receiver. 'Hi, Gina,' a voice says. But I'm not surprised that the man on the other end knows it is me and I say, 'Hi' back. We are chatting for a while, then the conversation turns to sex.

It doesn't seem uncomfortable for me to discuss it because I feel as if I know the caller already. He is telling me that I am the sexiest woman he has ever met and then goes on to describe our last lovemaking scene.

He describes how he undressed me as we were walking

up the stairs to my flat and that when we got inside the door, we were both practically naked. Passion overcame us and we ended up having sex on the carpet in the hallway.

As he is talking I feel myself getting very aroused and I undo my blouse and feel my left breast. The conversation gets steamier and steamier as he describes what we would both be doing if we were together now. I feel heady with desire. When he suggests we meet, I agree, but when I ask him where, the line goes crackle and his voice is faint. I am really annoyed because I wake up before I can make out what he is saying.

ANALYSIS

Gina is being very sensible by erring on the side of caution in meeting strange men. Dreams of telephones obviously relate to communication and exchange of information. On a practical level it could be seen that she is being ultra-safe, yet there could also be a message that there is in fact someone she has known for a long time who is trying to catch her eye. It could also be that someone from the past will pop up in her life again.

TOE-SUCKING

Fidelma recently split up with her husband after only three years of marriage. The split was acrimonious at first, with both of them blaming each other for the breakdown. But with hindsight they realise that they simply were not suited to each other and as a result their relationship is beginning to improve.

Recently, however, Fidelma has become involved with a man who works in the investment department of a large bank. Albert, her husband, is behaving as though he is jealous of the relationship and is always passing snide remarks about him to Fidelma. He is also beginning to mess her about over the divorce, by not replying to letters on time, losing important documents and cancelling meetings at the last minute.

THE DREAM

I am lying on a sun lounger with my eyes closed behind my sunglasses. I feel very relaxed. My husband is caressing my body with sun oil. He is enjoying rubbing it into my skin, perhaps too much really, as he is taking quite a long time to do it.

Every now and then he kisses me on a part of my body before he smoothes the oil over it. I sigh with relaxed contentment. Working down my legs, he kisses my thighs, then both my knees and my shins.

'I bet you wouldn't kiss my toes,' I say laughingly.

'Oh really?' he answers.

Moving his face to my feet, he kisses the top of them, then moves to the toes of my right foot and kisses every one of them — one by one. It's tickly and I squeal. Then, progressing to my left foot, he does the same again until he arrives at my big toe.

I can feel his warm mouth encircle it and at first I'm a bit taken aback, but I relax as he gently swirls his tongue around it. He playfully nips it but then the pressure increases and he is biting my toes hard. Energy drains from me and it is with great effort that I manage to pull my leg away. When I look at my toe, there is a river of blood coming from it. Then I wake up.

ANALYSIS
Fidelma's husband has got her exactly where he wants her, by the little 'piggies'. She is being drained of her resources by the divorce and the dream reflects this. What she needs to do is to gain a toe-hold on the situation and for that she needs to play as hard as he is doing. It may be worth her while getting a second legal opinion on her situation regarding the divorce.

Whatever happens she must grasp the situation, otherwise she will continue having to toe the line that her husband draws.

TONGUES

Sheila confided in a colleague a secret she had not told anyone at work: she had an abortion when she was just 17. She revealed her story during a heavy night on the town to celebrate their boss's birthday.

Now she regrets having said anything because the office she works in is always buzzing with gossip. She fears that she will become the target of their lunch-time natters. She is particularly worried because her boss is a devout Catholic and she thinks that if she hears about her past, she will make life difficult for her.

THE DREAM

I am in the shower at the gym with a group of colleagues. As I stand there facing the shower head and basking in the warmth of the water, I hear whispering behind me. It gets louder and louder as if there are a lot of people whispering. There is shampoo in my eyes, so when I turn around I can't open them and see who they are. Neither can I hear what they are discussing.

Once I rinse my face I can see the faces of people I know from my office. It's bizarre because they all have really long tongues and they are crowding around the shower cubicle. Their tongues get longer and longer and they start to flick them at me. Every now and then one of them touches my body and I recoil into the corner of the shower.

I feel really frightened by their presence and I lash out, trying to get them away from me. When I wake up I am thrashing around in bed and the dog is licking my face.

161

ANALYSIS

Often outside noises, touches and sensations are used in our dreams to represent something else. For example, an alarm clock going off could reveal itself in our dreams as a telephone ringing. There is an element of this in Sheila's dream, with the dog's licking triggering the tongue element in her dream.

However, she is also worried about having laid herself open to criticism and gossip when she bared her soul to a colleague. Hence the uncomfortable nakedness in the dream. It is always wise to try to hold your tongue in drink, but in practice it is very difficult.

The message that she can take from this dream is stop being paranoid about office gossip, and talk to her colleague again, ensuring that she keeps her confidence. If by chance her boss did find out, then if she was a true Catholic, she wouldn't pass judgment or throw the first stone at Sheila.

UNDERWATER SEX

Brian has always fancied himself as a bit of a playboy. He has dark, Italian looks that women go for and he knows that he is handsome. Unfortunately for the women he encounters, he is very fickle, always thinking that there is someone better out there for him. He couldn't be faithful to save his life.

But now the tables have been turned on him and he is not sure how to handle it. He met a woman who is just as good-looking as him and likewise knows it. Men flock around her, hanging on her every word. For the first time in his life, Brian has met his match, and he is smitten.

THE DREAM

I am swimming in the sea, aiming for some rocks that are jutting out. I want to get there, climb up and bask in the sun. I am getting a little tired the closer I get. I hear singing — it sounds so sweet — and then I see her: a mermaid. I remember thinking to myself, there is no such thing as a mermaid.

She slips into the water and swims over to me, taking me by the hand. We tread water and she kisses me. I feel dizzy and as my head is spinning, she pulls me out to sea, all the while smiling at me.

I feel compelled to follow. She dives deep into the water, still holding my hand. I manage to get a gulp of air before we submerge into the greeny depths.

Underwater her hair flows behind her body, which is half fish, half woman. Fascinated, I touch her and feel the most exquisite sense of ecstasy course through me.

On and on we swam in her underworld, all the while our bodies merging together. The water started to get darker and I began to feel apprehensive. She let go of my hand and all I could see was the silver flash of her tail as she disappeared into the murky depths. I started to panic. All around me the darkness closed in and I opened my mouth to scream, swallowing the cold, salty water. I couldn't find the surface and I woke up feeling as though I was drowning.

ANALYSIS

Water is a sensual substance, but it has hidden dangers, rather like Brian's new girlfriend. The tide has turned on him and he is out of his depth. The emotions he is experiencing are unknown to him. That is a good thing because for too long he has broken hearts. Now he is getting a dose of his own medicine and it's a bitter pill to swallow — like the salt sea water.

UNDERWEAR

Alan's son Joe has always been a quiet boy. He is very close to his mother and seems to prefer her company to his. As a child he was more interested in art than in playing boisterous games of football.

Alan never really took much notice until Joe reached his teenage years and always seemed to be hanging around with girls, rather than the boys. But even though he spent a lot of time with females, he never seemed to have any who were real girlfriends.

As any good father should do, Alan felt he ought to give Joe the 'bird and the bees' lesson. But when he tried to talk to Joe about it, the teenager dismissed him and told him he wasn't interested. This disturbed Alan but he is unsure why.

THE DREAM

About two nights after that conversation I had a dream about Joe. It strange because I never dream and I wish I hadn't had this one.

I arrive home from work earlier than expected. The house is quiet and because I feel unwell, I decide to lie down in bed for a while. I walk upstairs to my room, but decide to use the bathroom before I climb into bed. I try the handle but it's locked. I am puzzled because there isn't supposed to be anyone at home at this time. When I call out my wife's name there is no reply, then I call out Joe's.

I hear a lot of scuffling around and Joe answers, 'In a minute.' As I wait I go into my bedroom. My wife's underwear drawer is open and a selection of her bras are on the bed. That's weird, I think, because she is an extremely tidy person.

The bathroom door opens and almost immediately, my son's bedroom door closes. Just as I am about to walk into the bathroom, it dawns on me that my wife wouldn't have left the room in a mess. It must have been someone else.

I fling open the door of my son's bedroom, just in time to see him struggling to put on his bathrobe and wipe the lipstick off his face at the same time. He fails to cover up the ladies' underwear on time. I feel stunned and walk back across the landing. Then I wake up.

ANALYSIS

Alan is jumping to conclusions with regards to his son's sexuality. Teenagers are notoriously shy about discussing sex and often the last person they want to talk about it to is their parents.

While Alan thinks that Joe could be gay, it is a possibility that he has not aired with his son. He should think long and hard about his attitude towards homosexuality. It could be that Joe is gay, but Alan will never learn this from his son if the boy thinks he will react badly towards him.

Having thought honestly about his feelings on the subject, and his son's natural need of support at a difficult age, he should try again to talk to Joe.

VALENTINE

Fifteen-year-old Tracy has got a crush on her brother's friend, Craig. He is three years older than her and is unaware of her feelings. He sees her as just a kid. She tries to hang around in her brother's room, pretending to play records when they are both there.

Her brother thinks she's stupid and tries to get her out of the room. She hasn't told him what she thinks of Craig because she knows that he will make fun of her, but she would love to know what Craig thinks of her and if she has a chance with him.

THE DREAM

Sitting at my breakfast table are my family and me. I am eating cornflakes. The radio is on and the presenter is reading the news. There is a beautiful bunch of red roses in a glass vase on the table near the door. It is Valentine's Day and my father has bought them for my mother. The only card is one from him to her.

I am feeling very excited because the postman hasn't come yet and I am hoping that I get a card. I want it to be from Craig. The dog barks and the letterbox clicks open to the sound of something being pushed in. My brother jumps up and grabs the mail before I have a chance to make a move.

He holds a pink envelope high above his head, waving it around. 'Tracy's got a boyfriend,' he chants. I jump up to try to catch it but I can't reach. I am really frustrated and tears well in my eyes. My father sees I am getting upset and snatches the card out of my brother's hands.

I take it and run up to my bedroom, feverishly opening it as I go. It is a Valentine's card with two elephants on the front, but when I open it there is no writing inside — it is completely blank. Then I wake up.

ANALYSIS
This dream is a good omen, and Tracy will kiss someone in the future. It may not be Craig but it will be someone she likes. Teenagers often develop crushes and Tracy will have many more before she reaches adulthood. Perhaps Craig is a little old for her and she will find someone who is nearer her age. But she should continue to be friendly towards him, then maybe he will notice her some day.

VAMPIRE

Clive is a very unhappy man as he is caught between his wife and his mother. His wife is furious that his mother is constantly interfering with their lives and wants him to tell her to back off.

His mother, on the other hand, feels that his wife is selfish and that she, as a grandmother to his children, ought to have a say in their upbringing. The last time the family went around to his mother's for Sunday lunch, a huge row broke out over the table manners of one of his children. His wife walked out of the house after telling his mother she was 'an interfering old bat'.

Now ultimatums are being issued by both women and Clive doesn't know what to do.

THE DREAM
I am in bed with a very sexually experienced woman who knows just how to pleasure a man. She has lots of energy and she handles me expertly.

We are in the 69 position, both concentrating on each other's pleasure. Once I am spent and exhausted, she pulls out a scarf from a drawer and ties it around my head as a blindfold.

Then, taking a variety of things, she teases my body: first with what feels like a feather, then with ice. I never know where she is going to touch me next. Then she puts little kisses all around my neck, increasing the pressure so that they feel like love-bites.

As she becomes more passionate, she bites me harder. Now it's hurting and I pull off the blindfold and tell her to take it easy, but she ignores me. It takes me all my strength to push her off and when I do it gives me the fright of my life. She's a vampire, and her fangs are dripping with my blood. I was so horrified that I woke up with a start, sitting bolt upright in bed. I couldn't get back to sleep for ages.

ANALYSIS
The presence of vampires in a dream indicates that in waking time the dreamer is being drained of positive energy. They can also indicate that the dreamer is not receiving enough attention. Both are true in Clive's case. He needs to get the two women together and hold proper discussions about the problems, explaining to them how he feels about the situation. As long as he tries to placate them both, he is pleasing neither.

VIRGIN

Denise and Gary finally decided to tie the knot after a whirlwind romance of only three months. Her parents weren't too happy about it because they felt it took longer than that to see if a couple were right for each other for life. Her friends also think she is crazy but she has told them that she's only crazy about Gary.

They were due to marry within two months to coincide with her twenty-second birthday. Everything has been an absolute rush and she hasn't had time to think. Every time she and Gary talk, the main subject has been the wedding. Her big day finally arrived but she had a disturbing dream the night before.

THE DREAM
I am wearing a wedding dress, but it doesn't look like the one I bought. It is really lacy and fluffy. The wedding is over and I am standing in the bridal suite with my arms folded. I am even still wearing my veil.

Gary is talking but I can't hear what he is saying; he looks angry. When he goes to kiss me I turn away. 'I can't,' I say. 'I'm a virgin.'

He climbs into bed naked and looks at me, pulling back the covers and indicating that I should join him. I do, completely dressed. I lie there, still with my arms folded. Again he tries to kiss me, but I turn away and say, 'I can't. I'm a virgin.'

He turns over so that his back is towards me. I feel very scared and unhappy. It didn't help my mood first thing on my wedding day either.

171

ANALYSIS

Dreaming of being a virgin is an omen for the future. Marrying young and so quickly means that Denise and Gary have to get to know each other as a married couple. They have committed themselves to each other and will have to work at their relationship. There will be some disquiet in the future as they adjust to a new way of life, but if they are serious about each other they will work it out.

WATER SPORTS

Neil has been married to Zoe for seven years and during that time she has called the shots. She has always been a very dominating woman and now seems to be more opinionated than ever before. She decides where they go, what they eat, who they are friends with.

Now Neil has managed to get his own allotment plot and she is not happy about it. Every time he leaves the house to go to it, she throws a wobbly. More often than not he gives in to her because he can't stand the rows.

THE DREAM

My wife is coming up the garden path. She looks thunderous and when she gets to the front door she can't find her keys. She bangs on the door and calls my name. I come to the upstairs window above the door to answer her. She tells me not to be so stupid and to open the door.

When I tell her that I am desperate to go to the loo, she barks an order at me to do it now. I take her at her word and unzip my trousers and empty my bladder right on top of her. I laugh, but even though it's a sunny day, she has an umbrella and pulls it out of her bag. My urine bounces off the open umbrella and misses her completely.

I finish urinating and she looks up and snarls, 'Now open the door.' I feel really apprehensive and stand there wondering what I should do.

ANALYSIS

Dreaming of urinating is indicative of releasing tension

and emotional cleansing. Unfortunately for Neil, his efforts were in vain, because his wife thwarted him when she protected herself with the umbrella.

It is possible that Zoe may not realise that her behaviour is so destructive — after all, she has been allowed to behave as she likes for a long time. If Neil really can't bring himself to spell out his grievances forcefully and openly, then he should try putting his feelings in a letter at a time when he is going to be away for a while. It will give Zoe time to digest the contents and then they can talk about the problem when he returns.

YOUTHFUL SEX

Divorcee Alana was feeling very pleased with herself. After years of piling on the pounds she had managed to shed the excess two stone she had been carrying throughout her marriage to Giles.

It was only when her divorce came through that she realised that she still had a life to lead. It is a role she has thrown herself into with great energy. She is now a regular at the local aerobics classes and is making some new friends. Life is looking good for her now.

THE DREAM

I dream that I am at least 20 years younger than I am and full of life and energy. As I walk down the road men turn to look at me, and I feel radiant. I am on my way to meet my boyfriend at the local record store.

We meet up and we kiss, then clutching the records he bought, we go back to his bedsit. It's really cosy there and after downing our coffee, we start undressing each other.

I feel highly charged as we make love. The old iron bed creaks but I don't care who hears us — I just want to enjoy myself. We make love over and over again, never flagging and never feeling tired. The afternoon turns to dusk and then finally dark and we're still going. I wake up invigorated, but it doesn't mean I want a toyboy, does it?

ANALYSIS

You're as young as you feel, says the cliché. This seems to apply to Alana's situation, but more likely her dream is purely a reflection of the new energy she has attained recently. It's a good dream and people who dream of youth are usually young at heart.

ZOOPHILIA

James moved from London to South Wales, where he has a smallholding. It was the realisation of an ambition he had had for many years and he had been looking forward to the change in lifestyle.

He has a variety of animals, including pigs, goats and chickens. He and his girlfriend were keen to bring up their young son, Simon, in a better environment. They have been there for seven months and despite the odd problem, they have managed to be fairly self-sufficient. Everything seems to be working out nicely. However, there is a small fly in the ointment. Their neighbours have been very slow to get to know them and whenever James walks into the local pub some of the older residents start speaking in Welsh. He wants to become part of the local life, but feels they don't want to know.

THE DREAM

I am standing in a field full of sheep. The sky is a bright blue and the only sound I can hear is birdsong and the odd sheep baa.

There must be hundreds of sheep in that one field alone. I run after them and catch one, then I hold it while I unzip my trousers and prepare to have sex with it. It is bucking and jumping around, trying to escape, but I keep a tight hold on it.

I am concentrating so hard that I don't notice that the other sheep have clustered around me. When I look up, they have all got human faces which look accusingly at me. I feel terribly ashamed and guilty. I let go of the sheep and stand there exposed, with my wellington boots all covered in muck.

The sheep turn and surrounding my victim start to run across the field until they get to the farthest corner. They band together and watch me, not making a sound.

Then I wake up.

ANALYSIS

Whenever you have dreams in which animals play a big part, think of the qualities that these creatures are synonymous with. We all think of the sheep as being an animal that has a herd-like nature. The villagers in James's village have that kind of instinct. His approach to the sheep he was trying to have sex with is obviously wrong. The message that he can draw from the dream is twofold. First he should decide if his way of life is alienating the locals. Then he should consider whether compromising over his lifestyle is worth it if it means he and his family are not cold-shouldered by a group of people who obviously dislike change.

CHAPTER FOUR

TYPES OF DREAMS

This chapter looks at the major types of dream and the roles they play in your emotional life. Analysis of a dream is often helped by the ability to recognise it as belonging to a certain type, although, as we have seen, there are other important interpretative skills which must complement this categorisation.

CLEARING-HOUSE DREAMS

These could also be described as 'clutter dreams', for during them the mind reruns your experiences, almost always in a random order, as it sifts through mental and emotional furniture, acting just like a clearing-house.

Often, the mind seems to be racing as you first try to sleep and indeed the clearing-house dream is usually a baffling kaleidoscope of events and feelings. Some scientists believe it is simply a process whereby your mind sorts the wheat from the chaff, replaying then retaining important concerns and discarding useless ones.

Quiet focusing on the day's events, even meditation, immediately before sleep can help avoid this type of dream, which can leave you quite exhausted.

LUCID DREAMS

In the middle of a dream have you ever become consciously aware that you are — only dreaming? Have you ever experienced a 'false awakening' where you actually believe you have woken up only to find yourself still in your dream?

In so-called 'lucid dreams', the dreamer is aware that he or she is indeed dreaming. That can be either comforting, if the dream is one in which you are in some danger, or disturbing if you find yourself unable to wake up properly and are, in effect, trapped in a dream.

The term 'lucid dreaming' was first introduced into the language early this century by a Dutchman named van Eeden. It was considered to be so rare that even eminent psychiatrists interested in dream analysis dismissed it — until 73 per cent of people in a survey of a cross-section of society said they had experienced lucid dreams.

Tibetan Buddhists have developed techniques to promote lucid dreaming, believing it to be a true window on our inner souls. Dream analysts also assert that the experience of lucid dreaming — and, beyond that, the ability to control your thoughts while dreaming — can enhance an individual's intuition and imagination during their waking hours.

Further, some say the ability to lucid-dream can be learned, practised and even monitored. Leading proponent Stephen LaBerge, a university psychologist, has developed sensors which detect eye movements accompanying these most vivid of all dreams.

Indeed, lucid dreams can actually feel real, being accompanied by heightened senses of hearing, smell, taste and feeling. If you do lucid-dream regularly, experts suggest you can alter the circumstances of your dreams. Dream actions can be as simple as picking a flower or, for sexual dreamers, follow the advice of mystical Mexican Lothario Don Juan and try to look at your own hands in your dream.

OBSTACLE DREAMS

These dreams are about fear of failure or of fears that must be overcome before progress is possible. Unlike problem-solving dreams, they are far more complex in that the frightening dream itself may bear no relation to a deep-rooted real-life problem or phobia. For example, a dream in which you experience terror at the top of a wind-lashed skyscraper may mean you are full of trepidation about a recent promotion.

Common obstacle dreams include being lost in fog, being trapped in a walled enclosure, feeling threatened by hostile strangers or even being back in a school classroom staring at an exam paper, not a single question of which you can answer. All these dreams — and many more nightmares like them — can be deeply disturbing, yet they never point to the real dread of the dreamer. What they certainly signify, however, is that there is an obstacle in his or her waking life.

Dream symbols and dream analysis are dealt with elsewhere in this book and may be of help if you have a persistent obstacle dream.

OUTSIDE-INTERFERENCE DREAMS

These dreams are caused when anything in your physical environment causes enough disruption to invade your sleep. Such disturbances range from the sound of traffic outside your window to a buzzing fly in the bedroom to an icy feeling when the duvet falls to the floor or a pair of cold feet are pressing into you.

Similarly, falling asleep in front of the TV or while listening to the radio can cause any of the information you have been absorbing to invade your dream. During sleep, any sound or change of atmosphere whatsoever can have an effect on what you dream.

Such effects are, of course, meaningless; your dream is likely to be an unfathomable jumble, instantly forgettable when you wake and discover the cause of your disquiet. Obviously, the more tranquil the environment in which you sleep, the less likelihood there is of outside interference influencing your dreams.

There is, however, one potential danger signal which should not be ignored. A dream feeling of pain can mean that you are indeed physically suffering in some way. More often than not, you'll probably awake with nothing more worrying than a minor stomach ache or a headache but dream pains can signal a real problem.

PROBLEM-SOLVING DREAMS

These are dreams which give you answers to problems which, by day, may have puzzled and perplexed you, and indeed seem totally insoluble. They may be about work, home, even personal relationships, and often prove to be the most satisfying dreams of all, leading the dreamer to a positive conclusion or a fresh course of action.

As we sleep, our minds are unencumbered with day-to-day trivia, yet obviously retain all the knowledge and information that has been stored. Artists and scientists swear that apparently insurmountable problems have been solved, with crystal clarity, through dreams — almost as if the brain has been left in a state of uninterrupted peace to come up with an answer.

Try focusing your mind on a problem before you fall asleep. Don't fret or panic or desperately search your conscious mind for the answer; just focus calmly on the problem itself before you drift away into slumber. The dream solution that often results may not — indeed probably will not — be what you expected. But very often dreams will suggest a plan of action, or perhaps simply a different way of looking at a problem which then leads to a practical solution.

The problem, of course, doesn't have to be of a practical or even logical nature. How you feel about someone, a partner, say, can be a source of anxiety. How you dream about that person can perhaps help guide your future course, with — or without — them.

PROPHETIC DREAMS

These dreams, also referred to as 'precognitive', are glimpses into the future — windows on life to come. Precognition means foreknowing and many who have claimed to have had prophetic dreams must be treated with scepticism. There are, however, well-documented examples which defy any other explanation than that they were indeed truly prophetic.

Precognition differs from déjà vu in that it concerns someone other than yourself. Gurus, mystics and meditators have often claimed precognitive dream experiences and without doubt their dream-state minds are more open and attuned to psychic phenomena.

But ordinary individuals too have related dreams, about people and events of which they could have no prior knowledge, that have come true.

This account is not meant to cause alarm. Virtually all precognitive dreams are highly specific in detail, so that dreaming of an unidentifiable plane crashing the night before your flight is simply a reflection of your tension about travel.

TEACHING DREAMS

We all regularly have teaching dreams; they are the sleeping mind's way of preparing us for what lies ahead. Since most dreams reflect what we're currently involved in — at work, home and in relationships — the teaching version is an indicator of how to tackle the next stage of life.

Often, a déjà vu experience is the waking memory of what happened in the dream state, like when you just knew you were going to say or do something in a certain way or equally instinctively knew a certain person was going to respond to you or act in a certain way. In other words, the experience is a recall — usually a partial recall — of what you actually dreamed.

Teaching dreams themselves can take many forms; even the obvious classroom scenario with a favourite teacher from the dim and distant past imparting new wisdom is common.

Whatever the dream, though, the point is that it guides you in a particular way — guidance you may not even have been consciously aware you needed — unlike, for example, a problem-solving dream.

CHAPTER FIVE

COMMON DREAMS

SEASONAL DREAMS

The seasons have an undeniable effect on what we dream. In spring our dreams reflect growth and new beginnings, especially in women, for whom dreams of motherhood are common. Dreams at this time of the year will often deal with your emotional life and your relationships with others. It is a period, especially, for sexual dreams full of hope and promise.

Summer dreams are very often full of a carefree feeling, though problem-solving — even inventive or innovative — dreams are heightened during the summer months.

The dreams we have in autumn focus on the physical body, on sexuality and on creativity. There is a sense of completion about these dreams with their wealth of ideas and material things.

Dreams during the dark winter months are inward-looking, representing a time for self-appraisal and personal growth. During this cold season your dreams are at their clearest and most powerful and you are more likely to remember them than at any other time in the year.

There are many common themes which nearly everyone will encounter at one time or other in their dreams. But it must be remembered that these are merely common themes, and that fundamentally, every dream is unique to the person dreaming it. Therefore, when analysing a dream, take careful note of the symbolism of a dream, but tailor its interpretation to reflect your own life. Do not translate it literally.

There are very few people who have not experienced a falling dream or a chasing dream. However, the dream state throws up the most surprising subject-matter and the most incongruous situations. Dreams borrow symbolic behaviour and objects from all areas of our lives: from childhood, a passing conversation, or a long-forgotten incident. Even, it is thought, they borrow from genetic memory implanted in us by our ancestors dating back thousands of years.

The main point to remember about our dreams is that they can teach us something. Even our most horrific nightmares hold a message for us, and that is the great benefit of dreaming. Once we have learned to understand it we can take this information our dreams provide and act on it to create a better life.

BLOOD

To lose blood in a dream shows a loss of energy, vitality or virility. A bloody murder is indicative of killing off a part of oneself. Or it may be that you have a problem with your performance which is worrying you in your waking life. For example, as a singer, if you see blood coming from your throat, it may be a warning sign to take things easy or have a health check.

CHASE

You are running as hard as you can to get away from whatever is chasing you. You daren't look back because you are frightened of seeing something that you don't want to see. Instead you continue to run and your legs feel like lead; you feel as though you will never get away.

The truth is you won't, unless you turn around and face the monster.

The message from a dream like this is 'confront the fear'. By confronting it you will cause it to evaporate. At time of intense worry, particularly about finances, you will probably experience this type of dream. The anxiety of the day is trespassing into your night-time slumber to warn you – and on waking up you are exhausted.

Whatever you try to run away from, you will never achieve it because you are trying to run away from yourself. Make the peace and you will have a peaceful night.

DEATH

To dream of death is disturbing. But do not be frightened because out of death comes life. Death is merely part of the cycle of life. Death in a dream means the end of the old, to make way for the new. To see yourself dead in a dream is an encouraging sign as it also signifies the beginning of something new in your life. Seeing in your dream a person you knew but who is now dead could indicate that your emotions towards that person are dead and that you have very negative thoughts about them.

FALLING

You may find that you jerk awake, having dreamed that you are falling off a high building or even a chair. The drop seems endless but comes to a sudden halt. Some believe that we all leave our bodies at night and the falling sensation is connected with our rejoining into the body. A bad re-entry accounts for the falling sensation.

However, it is also thought that this sensation occurs during light sleep, just as you have fallen off to sleep. The interpretation of falling in a remembered dream is quite simple. Think of daily life — are you in control?

FLYING

To dream of flying can be great fun as it brings with it a sense of freedom and the feeling that anything can be achieved. You feel on top of the world and have an overview of everything that is going on.

But rather like falling, it is thought that the sensation of flying is brought about because the dreamer really can fly, by means of a process called astral projection. In some cases, dreamers are said to have travelled to foreign lands and brought back vivid memories of places they have never seen.

HOUSE

Houses with myriad rooms are among the most common elements in dreams. The events of such a dream take place in a variety of rooms. It is important to note where they occur because this has an over-riding influence on where the dreamer stands with a particular problem.

The house is symbolic of the dreamer. Different rooms represent different personal characteristics and doors open to reveal the different elements of our make-up. Thus windows are the opening to our soul. Moving upstairs to the bedrooms or attic show us rising to the heart of a problem.

SNAKES

The context in which a snake appears in a dream is important to note. Down the centuries snakes have been used to symbolise many things, from religious power to the physician's art to the phallus.

Snakes are synonymous with energy, passion and power. However, because of mankind's fear of the snake, we have always equated it with something that is not good, as in the story of Adam and Eve, where it represented the devil and temptation.

TEETH

Whoever dreams of loose teeth will without doubt be going through a time of turmoil in his or her relationships or working life. As we get older our bodies change, our skin becomes slacker, our bones more brittle and our teeth suffer from the wear and tear of preparing our food for digestion. Therefore the presence of teeth falling out in a dream represents inevitable change.

TOILET

Toilet dreams are associated with the inner emotions. They indicate how healthy our attitudes to these emotions are. If we are constipated, then obviously we are hung up on something emotional. All too often people let the past haunt their lives and carry around a load of crap — in addition to its literal meaning, we use the word to mean precisely that unwanted emotional baggage — that should have been dumped years ago. Whenever you have a dream about a toilet, on waking you should realise that it is indicative of your emotional state and that you need to address the situation.

TRAVEL

We travel to our destiny in life, whether by conscious thought or by fate. Travelling in our dreams shows us moving towards a destiny. Like houses, travel is one of the key dream elements. In our dreams, as in our daily lives, we travel by a variety of methods. The key to how well we are doing on our journey through life is to note the means by which we are travelling.

If it's a rocket, then we are destined for the dizzy heights of success. If we are on foot, then the journey will be long and tiring. But, whatever the mode of travel, if the dreamer stays the course, then he or she will reap the benefits of the journey.

WATER

Water in a dream is linked with the emotions. 'Still water runs deep' — how often have you heard that used to describe someone? Water in dreams conveys the state of our emotions, and like them it is susceptible to change. It takes only a mild wind to cause a ripple on a pond. The quality and clarity of the water is also important in order that you can look into it and see the message it holds.

Whenever water appears in your dream, think carefully about the state of your feelings.

This chapter offers you a useful A-Z directory of the most common dream symbols, including those with special sexual significance. The interpretations accompanying each symbol are designed to be a general guide. Use this directory in conjunction with the rest of the book, particularly Chapter 2, *Analysing Dreams*. This explains how to interpret your dreams, the meaning of which may depend on the interpretation of more than just one symbol.

CHAPTER SIX

COMMON DREAM SYMBOLS

A

Absurdity
If your dream is a mesmerising mish-mash of the absurd, making no sense whatsoever, take heart that it means you will find true happiness in love affairs, especially if the dream has a humourous twist.

Adam and Eve
Anyone dreaming of Adam and Eve in the Garden of Eden could be heading for trouble, not necessarily in a relationship. Such a dream can denote family, or perhaps health, problems ahead.

Adornment
Women who dream of dressing in beautiful clothes or wearing beautiful jewellery with the aim of impressing a male will have good fortune, not necessarily financially, but certainly in their love-lives.

Adultery
Dreams of adultery are almost always portents of distress or unhappiness but can ring a cautionary bell. If you dream, for example, of seeking an adulterous liaison, it may be warning you to choose new friends — or prospective partners — carefully.

Adventurer

Women can expect great passion from a handsome lover if they dream of an adventurous man. But men dreaming of an adventurous woman should beware; this dream means you will almost certainly have to prove yourself to a female in extremely delicate circumstances.

Advertisement

Dreaming of reading advertisements can mean two, opposite fortunes are in store. If the advertisements in your dream have pictures, prosperity is coming your way. If the ads have no pictures, hard work and a humble existence lie ahead.

Advice

If you dream of giving advice to a friend of a loved one you are likely to fall out with him or her. If, however, you dream of being given advice, look forward to happiness in love.

Aerial

If you dream of putting up an aerial of any sort it means a plan you thought was nearly impossible could be destined to come to fruition.

Affection

Any display of affection in a dream is a welcome symbol, denoting current happiness or foretelling a happy outcome to a love affair or marriage.

Age

Men beware! It's considered bad luck to dream of guessing a woman's age — it means there is a strong possibility of getting into trouble with someone of the opposite sex.

Agony
If you dream of suffering agony, you are likely to meet an old friend in need. To dream of someone else suffering means that a change of scene in some aspect of your life is possible. Dreaming of an animal in agony is a portent of terrible grief.

Air travel
Dreams of flying are normally not portents of free-spirited excitement to come. Instead they signify long periods of indecision in affairs of the heart.

Alcohol
If you dream of drinking in moderation, look forward to success. Anything more than moderation, especially drunkenness, warns of failure.

Alley
If you find yourself in a dark alley during a dream it can mean you are about to lose a lover. Arriving at the end of such an alley predicts the failure of a plan.

Allurement
In a dream, if you are aware of the attraction of a member of the opposite sex then be prepared to be the life and soul of the party, for an invitation is on its way to you.

Amazement
If you dream of being truly amazed or astonished, bank on an exciting experience in life soon.

Ambulance

This is a strong warning. If you see an ambulance in your dream the warning is against being indiscreet with a member of the opposite sex. If you dream of being in one, it is a more general caution against careless talk or rash behaviour.

Ambush

This is not a warning dream. However fretful you may feel after dreaming of being ambushed, be consoled that it simply means there is a pleasant surprise in store for you.

Anagram

A dream of playing or solving anagrams or word puzzles predicts a happy solution to difficulties in love.

Anchor

If you dream of anchoring a boat in harbour, you are set for a long, stress-free period in life. If you dream of raising the anchor, you are set fair for adventure. If you see the anchor from shore, a task will be successfully completed. When you see an anchor on ship, an opportunity is coming your way. To dream of an anchor dragging from the ship while you are on board predicts danger from an unknown source.

Anxiety

A feeling of anxiety in any dream, even if the source of the feeling is indiscernible, suggests loneliness.

Ape

If you dream of seeing an ape, someone is likely to make fun of you. If the ape chases you, you may lose your position at work through lack of care and attention.

Arrival
Arriving at a terminal means you are about to accomplish a difficult task. Seeing others arrive signifies good health.

Arrow
Any dreams of arrows should make you tread ultra-carefully in your love and sex life. To be hit by an arrow signifies disgrace, while shooting arrows at any kind of target indicates unfaithfulness.

Arson
If a man dreams of starting a fire the chances are that he is being warned against a woman in his life. Women who dream of committing arson are equally warned against a man with whom they are not yet close. A dream of seeing a fire being started by someone else is a portent of lost reputation.

Atlas
Journeys, long and short, are denoted by reading an atlas in your dream.

Attic
If you dream of rummaging around in an attic you have every chance of finding a loving mate and enjoying healthy children and worldly comfort. To dream of being a child playing in an attic is especially lucky.

Auction
Dreams of attending an auction denote that a pay rise or some other form of payment is coming your way.

Avalanche

Be extremely wary about health matters if you dream of an avalanche. Such a dream may signify physical illness or an on-coming disaster.

Axe

Dreaming of wielding a sharp axe is a portent of satisfaction. Women who have this dream can expect to meet a poor but honest lover.

B

Barriers
Fences, walls, closed doors and other barriers mean there are obstacles in your life which will thwart your plans.

Bay
Pleasure is in store for those who dream of sailing in a calm bay. But if the water is choppy, beware false friends.

Beach
You're lying naked on a beach in your dream and it feels like paradise. It won't quite be that when you wake — but you will be on the brink of a new and unusual course of action. If, in your dream, you are wearing a bathing suit it doesn't mean you're shy; just that you may have to explain something to someone close who has misunderstood you.

If you dream of dragging a boat up a beach it means you may be in need of financial help.

Bear
A bear's presence in a dream foretells fierce competition at work. Killing a bear signifies welcome freedom from a social commitment.

Beetle
If you dream of insects, especially beetles, crawling over your body, you are likely to face severe financial problems. If you kill the beetles, however, you will not only face but overcome such difficulties.

Bell

The sound of a bell tolling in a dream usually signifies the impending death of a distant friend or relative. Liberty bells, however, denote an upswing in the dreamer's business affairs.

Bench

If you dream of sitting on a bench, beware of trusting anyone who owes you money. If you simply see a bench in your dream, there is every chance of a reconciliation between you and a friend or loved one with whom you have argued.

Bereavement

Envisaging a death, especially that of a child, signifies failure. To dream of the death of a relative or friend foretells the frustration of plans and a bleak outlook for the future.

Bewitchment

Far from meaning a thrilling new encounter, when a man dreams of a totally bewitching woman he is destined for extreme financial problems.

Bickering

If you dream of bickering, nagging arguments, be prepared for just that in reality — a quarrel with a friend or someone you love.

Bird

One of the best omens for women is a dream of a bird or birds with beautiful plumage. For those seeking both love and wealth it can mean the ultimate prize — happy marriage to a wealthy man.

To catch a bird in your dream means good luck. But to kill a bird is a portent of disaster.

Dreaming of songless birds may signify that a crushing injustice is about to befall you.

Birth
Married women who dream of giving birth may not necessarily fall pregnant, for the dream more often predicts that money and happiness are to come.

Biscuits
Eating or baking biscuits can signify illness — or a family squabble over a trivial matter.

Blackbird
If you dream of a blackbird you may be called upon to show great courage in your life. If you dream of a dead blackbird be prepared for trouble.

Blackboard
To dream of a blackboard covered in white chalk writing means you are due to receive unhappy news of a friend.

Blemish
If a woman dreams she has one or more blemishes or spots on her face, she should not despair about her complexion. The dream simply means she will be wooed by many lovers.

Blindfold
Dreams of being blindfolded may herald disturbing influences in life. You may find yourself a victim of others' whims, or you may be the cause of someone else's distress.

Blindness
Often deeply disturbing, dreams of being blind can in fact foretell a possibly ruinous downturn in fortune. To see someone else blind means that someone is about to ask you for help.

Blonde
Blondes have more fun, the saying goes. Yet, in dream symbol terms, nothing could be further from the truth. Men who dream of blonde women are in danger, through illness, at home or at work. To dream of a blonde woman putting on a hat is a sign of a road accident.

Women who dream of being admired for having beautiful blonde hair are likely to suffer an illness.

Blossom
Seeing trees or shrubs in full flower in your dream heralds a period of prosperity and of peace of mind and body.

Blotting paper
The presence of blotting paper in a dream denotes a secret about to be betrayed, either by you or by someone else who could harm you.

Boasting
Don't feel proud of being a braggart in your dreams; boasting presages regret for an impulsive act which could cause trouble with a loved one or friend.

Boots
Dreaming of someone wearing boots can lead to a broken heart. Some dream analysts say that it means you are about to be replaced by someone else in the affections of

your partner or lover. If you are actually wearing the boots, new ones signify financial good fortune, while old ones spell sickness or trouble.

Box
Opening a box to find possessions or money signifies wealth and travel, but if the box is empty be prepared for a setback, usually in business.

Branch
Dreams of the branches of a tree waving in a gentle breeze signify fresh interests for anyone who has been finding life dull. If the tree is in bloom, those new interests will bring great comfort.

Bread
If you dream of eating bread your life may well be one of toil and worry on behalf of others, possibly troublesome children. If you see stale bread, unhappiness and illness could follow.

Breasts
Women who dream their breasts are sore are likely to face a real-life calamity, totally unconnected with their physical health yet deeply heart-wounding. Dreaming of flat or wrinkled breasts can also spell heartbreak to come. Female dreams of creamy, voluptuous breasts do not signal great passion — rather the possibility of great wealth.

Bride/Bridegroom/Bridesmaid
If a young woman dreams of being a bride it does not necessarily mean she will soon be walking down the aisle. Instead, it indicates she is due to inherit money. If a man

dreams of kissing a bride, it means he will be reconciled with former enemies, male or female.

A man who dreams of going through the wedding ceremony is likely soon to benefit from a financial windfall. If a man dreams of being nervous during the ceremony, he faces a momentous decision in real life.

If a woman dreams of being a bridesmaid, she is ready to wed. If her dress is torn in the dream, her husband will be secretive or furtive.

Bronze
If a woman dreams of a bronze statue, she will probably fail to marry the man of her choice. If the statue moves or even appears to be alive, she will fall deeply in love but will never wed. Dreaming of a bronze serpent or insect means you will face jealousy and insecurity.

Brothel
Far from the connotations being sleazy, if either a man or a woman dreams of visiting a brothel it signifies improvement in his or her life. It also signifies a happy, settled and comfortable home life.

Bugle
The resonant blast of a bugle in your dream portends unexpected happiness in your life — probably through someone far away. This is one of the better-known 'good luck' dream symbols.

Building
If the buildings in this frequent kind of dream are imposing or magnificent, you will be lucky with money and able to afford to travel to exotic locations. If they are modest

but well kept and clean, count on a happy home and work life. Unsightly, decaying old buildings, however, predict unhappiness.

Burial

If you dream of attending the funeral of a relative in the sunshine, be prepared for news that a family member plans to wed. If it's raining, brace yourself to learn that a relative is ill. A reversal of business fortune may also follow this dream.

If you experience the deeply disturbing nightmare of being buried alive means that you are on the brink of making a serious mistake.

Butterfly

A butterfly fluttering through your dream is always an omen of good fortune — especially for women, for whom it may foretell an early marriage to a handsome and virile man.

C

Camera

If you dream of taking photographs with a camera, beware of gossips who might do you down. If the pictures are moving, as if taken by a cine camera or camcorder, you will find it more difficult to rise above the scandal or disgrace your gossiping detractors are causing.

Cat

Normally, dreaming of a cat means bad luck, unless you chase it away. Seeing a cat asleep in a chair, though, has special significance for lovers. This symbol means the dreamer can look forward to a true sexual awakening, for the slumbering feline denotes great gratification from your love-life. If you hear the cat miaowing in your dream, it means that someone is speaking ill of you and damaging your reputation. If a cat scratches you, an enemy will try to cheat you.

Catastrophe

If a nightmare leads you to witness or be involved in a catastrophe, fear not. It simply signifies there will be a major upheaval in your life, but not necessarily to your detriment.

Cave

If you dream of seeing the entrance to a dark cave by moonlight, beware; your business and health could be in danger. If a woman dreams of entering a cave with a man, it means she will fall for a rogue, possibly even a crook, and stands to lose many of her friends as a result. If, however, she dreams of being captured and dragged into the cave by a caveman it means, ironically, that she can look forward to future happiness in married life.

Celibacy
Strangely, dreams of being celibate have no sexual connotation whatsoever. They simply mean that you will fail to accomplish something close to your heart.

Cellar
If you dream of a gloomy, musty cellar the chances are you face depression or even fear in life. This dream can be especially ominous for women, as it means they are likely to have an affair with a shady, untrustworthy man.

Cemetery
To dream of an ill-kept, desolate cemetery means you will outlive all your relatives and spend your final years alone among strangers. But if the graveyard is beautiful, you are assured happiness.

If a woman dreams of passing a cemetery on her way to her wedding, it means that she will outlive her husband or her husband-to-be.

Dreams of young children playing among gravestones denote a happy and healthy future.

Choir
Dream of singing in a choir and your waking endeavours are likely soon to be rewarded with some honour or prize. If you dream of singing a solo part, it means that your love-life will flourish.

Christmas

Dreaming of Christmas — white or otherwise — foretells prosperity, happiness and peace.

Circle

If you dream of drawing a perfect circle, either freehand or with compasses, you will see your plans and ambitions come to fruition.

Classroom

The romantic interpretation of this dream is the same for both men and women; if you imagine yourself in a school classroom, your likely partner in love will be someone you have known since your childhood, possibly an old school friend.

Clock

Most dreams of clocks are about decision-making. If you hear a clock ticking, you should not be wasting time on trivial matters. If you hear a clock strike, it means someone is waiting, impatiently perhaps, for you to make an important decision.If you wind a clock in your dream, you will find lasting happiness in love.

Coal

Dreaming of coal should make you a merry soul. If you dream of buying it, your income could be as much as doubled within the next few weeks. Putting coal on a fire signifies business success while delivering it predicts you are due to climb the social ladder.

Dreaming of a coal mine heralds a pay rise for anyone engaged in manual labour.

Cock crow

Hearing a cock crowing in your dream means you are about to make a lucky discovery.

Combing

Anyone who dreams of combing their hair will find the solution to a long-term problem. Men who dream of combing women's hair, though, should take it as a warning against pursuing a current flirtation too far.

Cosmetics

Many women dream of putting on cosmetics and the dream augurs well if the make-up is being applied in private. Should a woman dream of putting on lipstick, eyeshadow or other make-up in public, it signals the end of a romance.

Men dreaming of women applying make-up face trouble at work.

Cottage

Young lovers, in particular, dream of living in an idyllic country cottage. It's a comforting dream and so it should be, for it means that married life is likely to be blissful. If there is a vine on the cottage, there will be happy, healthy children to bless the union.

Cow

A woman who dreams of a herd of cattle will find true romance, happiness and contentment in the arms of her lover. However, if the dream is of cows that are difficult to milk, you will lose your sweetheart because of your coldness or indifference.

In general terms, stampeding cattle mean you will

accrue wealth, underfed cattle mean you are destined to a life of hard toil, and healthy, well-fed cows indicate that you are destined for happy times.

Cowardice
To dream of being a coward predicts the very reverse; in a real-life situation soon you will be brave and bold.

Crab
Dream lovers be warned! If you dream of fishing for crabs, a member of the opposite sex is out to get their claws into you — and they don't have honourable motives. The dream should caution you against a would-be lover or partner who is only interested in using you.

To dream of cooking crabs predicts a slight accident. To dream of eating them augurs good luck at gambling.

Cream
A woman who dreams of skimming the cream from the top of the milk will have many lovers but settle with, and only truly love, one husband.

Creek
If you dream of swimming in a creek your love, sex and work life will be hugely enhanced. This is a dream which indicates extraordinary luck in everything you do.

Crocodile
Great fortune follows a dream of being chased by a crocodile. If the creature catches you, however, you are facing a painful accident. But if you elude the crocodile, you may expect success beyond your wildest expectations.

Crown

It's extremely bad luck to dream of wearing a crown, even in a party or playful dream scenario. This dream means that you will be sorely tempted — and are likely to succumb to that temptation.

Cucumber

Eating a cucumber in a dream is a terrible portent of death in the family. If you dream of cooking a cucumber be prepared for rotten luck in business.

Cuddling

Contrary to what you might imagine, cuddling in your dreams carries a warning. Curling up with your loved one is actually a caution against promiscuity. While the dream may seem cosy and tame, it's a portent of naughty but not-so-nice things to come.

Curtain

Raising a curtain means you'll succeed in the enterprise which interests you most. Lowering a curtain means the exact opposite. If a curtain suddenly snaps open while either opening or closing, expect surprising news.

D

Dagger
If you dream of seeing a dagger, beware of enemies, either current or potential. This dream almost certainly means you will become embroiled in an unpleasant — perhaps dangerous — incident.

To dream of seeing someone stabbed by a dagger means you will overcome opposition, but you are still warned to act with caution in future dealings with others.

Daisy
For a man to dream of daisies doesn't mean he is a pansy. However cynical you may be, dreaming of daisies is very common for both sexes. Dream of a white daisy and your love will be true to you, while if you dream of a yellow one it means beware of a rival.

Dam
Dreaming of seeing turbulent waters rushing over a dam is a truly bad omen. Any deal in the offing is doomed to failure if you have this dream. But if you see a dam across a calm watercourse and the sun is shining, the reverse is true; you're in for good luck.

Dancing
Being young and dreaming of dancing the night away with someone of the opposite sex means that you can look forward to a joyous conclusion to your love affair.

If you're married and dream of dancing, the future holds happiness and bright, healthy children.

Dangling

If you dream that you are dangling from on high, beware of business dealings. This dream is telling you: 'Look before you leap.'

Darkness

If you dream that the day suddenly grows dark, or that there is an unexpected eclipse of the sun or moon, then what may transpire is beyond the realms of normal experience. Such dreams presage supernatural or perhaps telepathic experiences. What may be inexplicable in your dream could lead to an incident beyond explanation in your waking life.

Dawn

Dreams of the rising sun herald a new dawn in your life, and should be treated as foretelling brilliant opportunities to better your prospects. If, however, the day dawns grey, with threatening rain, you will come a cropper in a big deal or project in which you have been involved.

A dream of seeing the day break after a long, dark night signals new hope or new beginnings after a period of illness, distress or depression.

Daze

Dreaming that you are walking around in a daze means that others are spreading scurrilous rumours or gossip about you.

Deafness

Surprisingly, to dream of being afflicted by deafness actually means a happy solution to any day-to-day problems you may have.

Debauchery

Dreams of wanton debauchery may be deeply sexually gratifying. However, they really mean impending domestic doom or, for those who are single, warn against getting involved with anyone who sleeps around.

Deck

Lovers who dream of being together on the deck of a large ocean liner are destined for good luck. Whether you stand, sit or lie on the deck of any ship in motion, you are in line for good fortune.

Deer

Dreams of a deer, however elegant, normally signify a coming war. This can mean a bust-up with family or friends, being summoned to court or any other confrontation. Conversely, for lovers, dream visions of deer or fawns denote deep and lasting affection and possibly early marriage. If a young man or woman dreams of killing a deer, then a broken engagement is in the offing.

Despair

If you dream of being in despair through danger, lack of money or any other fraught situation, do not abandon hope. This dream means your fortunes are about to enjoy an upswing.

Divorce

If you are married, dreaming of divorce carries an obvious message: mend your relationship with your loved one before it's too late.

If you're single, sadly the dream means that your current affair is doomed to failure.

Dragon

This fiery beast of mythology shouldn't scare you; dreams of dragons either portend great riches and fortunes to come or prophesy meeting someone, possibly royal, who enjoys great fame.

Drain

Dreams of drains foretell sickness and should prompt the dreamer to try to stay fit and enjoy as much sunshine as possible.

Drool

Dream of drooling like a baby and you're not hungry for food or even love. You will, however, enjoy good times with a group of young people.

Drowning

Dreaming of drowning forewarns of bitter sorrow to follow in real life.

Dungeon

Some analysts say this is a symbol of envy. Yet the classic definition is that dreaming of a dungeon means you are due to be visited by a wealthy relative who you do not admire or respect.

Dwarf

Dream of a dwarf and you'll be healthy, wealthy and wise. It will be as if your problems have disappeared by magic. This is truly one of the luckiest dreams of all.

Dynamite

If you dream of seeing something blown up, your latest

plans will go awry. If you envisage dynamite — or any other explosives — being loaded on board a ship or any other vehicle then a danger to which you have recently been exposed is over.

E

Eagle
Seeing an eagle soaring on high is always a favourable dream symbol. Most often it signifies good prospects at work, though it can also mean the return of a friend from whom you have been separated. If, however, you dream of being carried away by an eagle, it can be a portent of bad health. Worse still, an eagle landing on your head symbolises death.

Ear/Ear-rings
If you dream of ears expect startling news in the post. Dream of touching or pulling someone's ear and be prepared for a bust-up with your boss at work. Men who dream of seeing an attractive woman wearing ear-rings are about to embark on a wild affair with an adventurous woman who leads all her lovers a merry dance before leaving them regretting the entanglement.

Earthquake
Witnessing the horrors of an earthquake in a dream means that some aspect of your life, usually work or business, is about to crumble. But take heart: you will survive and not only recover from the difficulties you experience but thrive as never before.

Eating
Dreaming of dining with guests signals good luck and happy times. However, dreams of eating alone can be a portent of misfortune.

Echo

If you dream of hearing the echo of your own voice, get set for an offbeat, possibly even bizarre, experience with a member of the opposite sex.

Eclipse

Dreaming of an eclipse of the sun or moon denotes a fear of an impending tragedy which would afflict yourself or an immediate member of your family .

Ecstasy

Love and sexual joy are yours if you dream of feeling as if you are in a state of ecstasy. This dream can signify a proposal of marriage or the acceptance of your hand if you are the proposer. If you dream of being in ecstasy while dancing, be prepared for a sizzling romance with a new lover.

Editor

Dreaming of an editor at his or her desk is a warning to check your accounts and balance your budget. Dreaming of being an editor means you are feeling unhappy with your lot in life.

Egg

Any sort of egg in a dream augurs well, indicating success in any new venture. Eating eggs speaks of excellent health in the future.

Elephant

All dreams about elephants are lucky. Seeing elephants performing tricks means a happy family life. Seeing them at work as a herd means good business prospects.

Enemy

To dream of overcoming an enemy is a good sign. Dreaming that an enemy gets the better of you in some way, is a warning of danger to come.

Engagement

Dream of being engaged and you may be disappointed, for it can mean that you will always be celibate.

Entombment

It may be disturbing to dream that you are entombed. Yet this is no more than a gentle warning to relax more and cease worrying about the impression you make on others.

Envy

Feeling jealous of someone's possessions in a dream is an omen that your own fortunes will take a turn for the better. If you dream of envying someone else's looks, though, your relationship will be rocked by bad temper, which could leave both parties miserable.

Equator

Crossing the equator in a dream does not denote travel to exotic places. Rather it means you are unsettled and indecisive and carefully need to consider current actions and relationships. If you approach the equator but do not cross it, you are likely to rue a lost opportunity.

Escalator

Ascending escalators mean new friends, new places, new hopes and ambitions. A descending escalator means a probable defeat, which you will have a struggle to turn into success.

Escape

Any dream in which you escape from any kind of peril suggests speedy recovery from what threatens to be serious illness. If you dream of someone else escaping from any soft of disaster, expect a cheque in the post soon.

Evening

If you dream of a balmy summer's night illuminated by the stars, you are destined to fall in love at first sight. If you dream of seeing a star and making a wish, look forward to happiness and a rosy, contented future.

Evil spirits

Nightmares about the presence of evil spirits mean you will be thwarted in current ambitions, although you will find peace and happiness on another course in life. If those spirits are close to you in your dream and resemble hideous faces that appear and disappear, you are likely to encounter new situations that will mystify you and cause confusion.

Execution

If you dream of being executed by any method — it is most likely to be by hanging, firing squad or electrocution — take good care of your health, for a long period of illness may follow.

Explosion

If you dream of witnessing any form of explosion in your dream, you are destined for a permanent improvement in both health and finances. However, if you witness a gun being fired, causing someone to be killed, the exact opposite is the case.

Eye/Eyebrow/Eyelash

Floating eyes, unattached to a face, are a symbol of money coming your way. To dream of a face with heavy or bushy eyebrows means you will be held in high esteem by all. A thick, heavily arched eyebrow is known as a mandarin eyebrow and denotes aristocracy and a cultured background. If, however, the eyebrows are thin and weak on your dream face, be prepared for failure both at work and in your love-life. Long, silky eyelashes predict that you will soon be sharing a secret which may disturb you.

F

Face
Very often, faces in dreams are unknown to the dreamer. The appearance of a dream face can have many, complex meanings and here is a brief guide.

A happy, smiling face means you are about to meet new friends and enjoy new pleasures in life. Faces which at first may appear to be friendly but then grow ugly or distorted portend disaster and possible death. To wash your face and dry it with a clean towel means that you will repent an action of which you are ashamed. Seeing a black face signifies a long life. Faces that snarl or grimace at you denote a quarrel with a loved one. Sadly, if you dream of seeing your own face, the prediction is one of great unhappiness or impending tragedy.

Facial
Women who dream of having a facial at a beauty parlour may have a guilty secret. This dream signifies a feeling of selfishness, accompanied perhaps by a sense of guilt.

Factory
To dream of a factory full of busy, bustling and happy workers is an excellent omen for business prospects. To dream of working in a factory does not mean you are destined for a life on the production line; rather, it signifies that your endeavours in life will reap their just reward.

Failure
Lovers who dream of proposing to, but being rejected by, their partners should take comfort. This dream is a

reminder to pursue keenly the object of your desire. If you do, he or she will almost certainly fall into your arms for keeps. To dream of failure at work should ensure the opposite: complete success.

Fainting
A man who dreams of rushing to the aid of a beautiful girl who has fainted should beware of a scheming woman who may have intentions other than love. If you dream of fainting yourself, treat this as a warning against possibly frivolous ways or dubious friends.

Fairy
Fairies, pixies, elves and all those other quaint creatures from children's books mean that you will have a golden opportunity of making a young person happy. If you dream of being one of those fictitious creatures, beware the way you behave in public, for your actions may be misconstrued by others.

Falcon
The falcon is a fairly common dream symbol. If you dream of seeing one poised for flight, it means that the decisions you make and your actions in life are likely to be honourable. If you dream of hunting with a falcon on your arm, beware of thieves. If a young woman dreams of a falcon, it means her romantic desires will almost certainly be fulfilled, though she is likely to have a rival for the affections of another.

Fame
If you dream of being famous, get set for a rough ride. This dream signifies a distinct turn for the worse in your

personal affairs. If you dream of seeing or meeting a famous person, it means help is coming your way from an unexpected quarter.

Family
To see a large and happy family in your dream suggests that you will spend a holiday abroad alone. To see a family of animals suckling at their mother's breasts suggests an upswing in your working life.

Famine
Dreaming of a country in the desperate throes of famine predicts an unsettled period in life during which you will suffer but eventually overcome all problems.

Fan
If a man dreams of a pretty girl fanning herself, jealousy and possibly even a broken engagement are imminent. To fan yourself means that a romantic liaison is proving too tangled and complex for you to cope with. To dream of losing a fan means that your lover's passion has gone cold.

Fanfare
If, in your dreams, you are greeted by a fanfare of trumpets, be warned that someone is hell-bent on ridiculing you or doing you harm.

Father
If you dream of your own father, be prepared for a possible change of environment. This can be as extreme as a city dweller moving to the country or vice versa. If you dream of being a father, perhaps surrounded by children, it heralds improving fortunes and possibly

a beneficial change of job.

Fatness
Fear not if you dream of being very fat and uncomfortable; you will have many friends and few worries.

Feather
If you dream of a cloud of feathers in the air, as though from a burst pillow, you are set for outstanding success which will make you proud as well as richer. Dreaming of eagle feathers predicts success and realisation of your ambitions; ostrich feathers signify the clinching of a deal.

Fence
If you dream of building a fence you are destined to be truly lucky in love. But if the fence falls down, you will lose your lover or partner. To dream of climbing a fence means you will realise your ambitions in full.

Dreams of the other type of fence — a dealer in stolen goods — portend failure in business.

Ferret
Dreaming of a furry little ferret is a harbinger of either disease or severe illness in your family or circle of friends.

Festival
If you dream of attending any sort of public festival, you will be happy at the good fortune of a friend.

Fever
If, in your dream, you have a fever or a running a high temperature, be prepared for a bumpy ride in your love-life. This dream means your relationship with your partner is

likely to take a sudden, unwelcome turn for the worse.

Fighting cock
If you dream of a contest between fighting cocks, beware of someone envious who is trying to wrest your possessions away from you.

Fighting
If you dream of being in a fist-fight, it means that, far from being aggressive by nature, you will be highly regarded by other people.

Filing cabinet
Unless you are searching for a lost letter, working at a filing cabinet signifies good luck. However, if you are searching for a lost letter, learn to keep yourself in check; this dream means a lowering of moral standards.

Finger/Fingernail
Blowing a kiss from your fingers to someone of the opposite sex means your love life will be exciting. To point a finger scornfully means you are losing someone's respect. If a woman dreams of polishing her fingernails, others are likely to be highly critical of her behaviour.

Fire engine
Dreaming of a fire engine normally heralds extremely good financial luck. To be at the scene of an inferno and see the fire engine leaving is luckier still.

Fire
It is a sign of bad luck if you dream of being burned. But if the fire gives you warmth and comfort, the exact oppo-

site is true. Dreaming of building a fire means an exciting sexual adventure is on the cards. Looking at a building which is ablaze means that soon someone will be seeking your health or sympathy.

Fire-fighter
A man who dreams of being a fire-fighter can expect an invitation to a stag party where there are likely to be some highly influential guests. If you dream of driving a fire engine, you are likely to have a narrow escape from an accident.

Fireplace
Home comforts are yours if you dream of sitting in front of a fireplace in which a roaring fire is keeping you warm. If there is no fire in the hearth, however, be prepared for a major upset in your love-life.

Fireworks
Sorry, but life isn't going to go with a bang if you dream of rockets, bangers, Catherine wheels or indeed any other fireworks lighting up the night sky. Rather, this dream indicates failure in a task you have set yourself.

Flatulence
Breaking wind in the company of others in your dream means you are bound for a serious bust-up with someone at work. If you dream of someone else breaking wind, pack your bags in preparation for a long journey.

Flower
Good luck follows any dream about almost any garden flower. Dreams of wild flowers prophesy adventure and

excitement to come, possibly in a new, wild romance.

Flute
The sweet music of a flute in your dream signals peace and contentment in family life. However, if you dream of playing the instrument yourself, beware of being caught in an embarrassing situation.

Flying
If you dream of being able to fly like a bird you may be, in your waking life, attempting the impossible. However, if the dream is of an aeroplane in flight, the omen is one of good luck.

Fork
Dreams of eating with a fork indicate relief from pain. But if you dream of stabbing someone with a fork, it indicates a loss of position.

Fortune-telling
Having your fortune told in a dream points to a wildly successful love and sex life — even if the fortune told in your dream is not good.

Fountain
Dreams of fountains suggest a happy and contented married life. If the fountain is dry, though, be prepared for a period of frustration in life.

Fox
A fox in your dream is a clear warning to beware of someone who intends you harm.

Frog

Dreaming of a frog is an omen of peace, tranquillity and restfulness in your life. To hear one croak means you will progress steadily at work and at home. If you dream of eating frogs' legs, close friends are likely to love and understand you deeply.

Fruit

Dreams of ripe fruit indicate good health. If the fruit is unripe, the reverse is true.

Fur

A woman who dreams of dressing in a luxurious fur coat is destined for doom-laden relationships with men. If, however, the fur is worn and tatty, she will be showered with honours and accolades. A man who dreams of wearing a fur overcoat can look foward to a long period of prosperity.

Fury

To dream of being in a rage predicts an action which will make you look foolish or ridiculous. If you dream that someone else is furious, watch carefully the behaviour of any friends or companions whose actions may be wayward.

G

Gale
Dreams of witnessing, or being trapped in, a ferocious gale signify a potential series of misfortunes. You may be aware that some of these are imminent and this dream should serve as a warning to watch every step you take, especially in financial matters.

Galleon
Dreams of a traditional Spanish galleon signify escape or release. For example, if you've felt trapped in a relationship which clearly isn't going to work, this dream means that you are on the brink of finding a way out.

Gallows
Lovers beware! A dream in which you see the hangman's gallows means a marriage, engagement or other relationship is doomed. If the dream turns into a terrible nightmare in which you see a victim hanging from the gallows, then you will have to overcome an enormous obstacle before you can find true happiness.

Garden
Any dream of a beautiful garden is a tremendously good omen for both sexes, symbolising love, happiness and even spiritual fulfilment. If the dream is of an unkempt garden, however, the reverse is true.

Gas
If you dream of smelling leaking gas, treat it as a warning not to interfere or meddle in other people's affairs. To

dream of seeing a victim overcome by gas foretells the possibility of a scandal, so beware of any indiscretions in your love life.

Gate
If you dream of coming to an open gate, opportunities in all areas of your life are about to open up invitingly. If the gate is closed, hopes you may have had are likely to be dashed.

Gift
If you dream of receiving any sort of gift, unexpected pleasures lie ahead, especially in your relationship with someone close. To dream of offering a gift means you may have heavy responsibilities, especially towards one you love, but you shoulder them happily.

Girl
When a man dreams of a pretty girl, the symbol of love shines bright over his life. This doesn't mean, of course, that the girl he loves or is destined to fall in love with is necessarily pretty herself. Nor does it mean that the course of true love will not be without pitfalls. Yet it remains the strongest dream indication of all for any male that he has found or will find love.

If a man dreams of a plain girl, it can mean the affection he offers will be rejected.

Glass
The expression 'walking on broken glass' could not be more appropriate than when used of any dream involving glass. Such a dream means you are about to have a sharp argument with the one you love. If it is to be short as well

as sharp, and not cause any lasting harm, is up to you. To dream of breaking glass indicates a radical change in your life — one you will be powerless to resist. To dream of putting glass into a window frame, however, is a sign of contentment at home.

Gold
Dreaming of gold indicates greed and warns you that this vice may cost you the affection of someone close. If you dream of digging for, or mining, gold, then you are dissatisfied with your home life.

Goose
Seeing a goose is not an encouraging dream, especially for women, for it means you must watch the scales, lose weight or alter your diet.

Gorilla
If you dream of being stalked by a wild gorilla, you are concealing a major embarrassment, the possible exposure of which haunts you. Beware of public humiliation.

Gown
Women who dream of wearing an elegant ballgown yearn to be the centre of attention. This dream means that this desire is often fulfilled, though not necessarily to the dreamer's entire satisfaction.

Grandparent
If you dream of your grandfather, expect acclaim from work or the community in which you live. If you dream of your grandmother, good luck is in store.

Grape

A dream of picking or eating grapes means your career is scaling new heights. Get set for promotion and the financial rewards that go with it.

Grass

Sexual joy and money are yours if you dream of grass bordering a flower bed. If the grass in your dream is brown, neglected or gone to seed, then you will have to work very hard both in love and in your financial dealings to get what you want.

Grasshopper

Dreaming of a grasshopper augurs uncertain times ahead. Take advice from one you love and trust to overcome what seem to be bewildering times.

Guillotine

Nightmares which focus on the guillotine can have a terrible bearing on your real life. If you dream of seeing someone brought to the guillotine for execution, it indicates that you will have a serious bust-up with a friend. If you see yourself as the victim, serious — even fatal — illness is in the offing.

Guitar

The sound of a guitar in your dream is likely to awaken your love-life. Gentle plucking on this instrument means that, whether you yet realise it or not, you are about to embark on a wonderful relationship. However, it is a more negative indication if you dream of playing the guitar yourself, for someone may be taking you for a ride and could let you down.

Gymnasium

Dreams of working out in the gym do not indicate that your health and fitness are on the upswing. But they do mean that you are becoming more outward-going and so are likely to receive many more social invitations.

H

Hair

In many manifestations, this is one of the most common dreams of all. If you dream of combing the hair of a member of the opposite sex, any sexual problems you may have with your partner will soon be solved. If you dream of combing the hair of a person of the same sex, the chances are you are worried about a friend in need, and your subconscious is letting you know you have the ability to help.

If you dream of having your hair cut, you are prepared for and sure to be successful in a new venture in life. If you dream of cutting someone else's hair, be warned about a supposed friend who may be seeking to do you harm.

If a woman dreams of having her hair permed, she is on the brink of an exciting new relationship with a man. If, however, a man dreams of having his hair permed, he is hiding a guilty secret and could risk facing shame and scorn from a lover or friends.

Hairdresser

Women who imagine being at the hairdresser's in their dreams should guard against repeating any scurrilous gossip they may have heard.

Halo

This dream is a bad omen. If you see someone with a halo, a friend is in grave danger. If an acquaintance has a halo, there could be an imminent death in the family. But if you see yourself wearing a halo in your dream, the only portent is that you are likely soon to face a long journey.

Hammer
Using a hammer for any purpose in your dream suggests success and achievement for women but failure or an accident for men.

Hammock
If you dream of reclining in a hammock with someone of the opposite sex, your love-life is likely to go with a swing too. If you're alone, the dream is telling you that your behaviour of late may be selfish, leading to irritations in life that you can nevertheless easily abolish.

Hand
Busy, skilful hands in your dream suggest that you enjoy working hard then playing hard too. No harm in that. Nor is there in a dream of beautiful hands, signifying satisfaction with life. A dream of gnarled, bent hands is also a good omen, suggesting you are on the verge of finding a way out of current financial problems.

Handbag
You're facing a mystery in life if you dream of a handbag. If you see someone searching through a handbag, a situation is in the offing which calls for your deep understanding and sympathy.

Handicap
To succeed in a dream despite any sort of handicap is a sign that in life too you will be successful, especially in your work.

Hanging/Hangman
To be present at a hanging, as well as suggesting a great

obstacle to be overcome, can mean that you are being called upon to cover up for someone or give an alibi of some sort. Worry if you dream of being a hangman; it is a warning against being too critical of loved ones or friends (*see also* Gallows).

Harbour

To dream of entering a harbour by ship suggests that success is in sight for a plan you may have. Leaving a harbour means you are planning a journey.

Harem

A woman who dreams of belonging to a harem is prone to upsets in her love-life and should heed the dream as a warning to pay greater attention to her lover. A man who dreams of keeping a harem fears — and may face — scorn from others.

Harlot

Far from being a scarlet woman herself, any woman who dreams of being a harlot is expecting good news from some source. If a man dreams of harlots, however, he should be warned that his health is failing (*see also* Prostitute, Prostitution).

Hate

Life is sad for you and will more than likely continue to be so if you dream of hating someone. If you dream that someone hates you, though, it is an omen of good luck coming your way.

History

Famous historical events signal an opportunity on the

horizon, so treat this as an appeal for you to be prepared.

Home
If you dream of a happy home life, this mirrors a contentment with your everyday life that is set to continue.

Honeymoon
If a man or woman dreams of being on his or her honeymoon, then the dreamer is ready for wedlock, either with a current partner or a lover yet to be discovered.

Honeysuckle
The sight or sweet scent of honeysuckle in a dream is an omen that true love is within reach to anyone searching for a partner.

Hoof
Seeing the hoof of a cow, horse or any other animal in a dream means you are in danger — or at least fear you are — of being swindled by someone. If a lover dreams of a cloven hoof, then the dream means there may be complications in the relationship which will be difficult to overcome.

Horse
A horse is a very common dream symbol, with several different connotations. In general, dreaming of a horse or horses suggests that you feel those around you are being faithful. If you dream of riding a horse, you feel capable of great achievement and the future augurs well. If you dream of training a horse, you may be experiencing resistance from someone you long to be closer to but who you feel doesn't yet fully trust you. If you dream of being

kicked by a horse, this is a warning against overconfidence in your dealings with others and the trust you freely give them. Seeing two horses fight in a dream could mean you face misfortune through complacency or misplaced trust.

If you ride a horse in your dream you will reap the rewards of someone else's endeavours.

Hotel

Sadly, this is not always a portent of a romantic weekend with your lover. If you dream of checking into an hotel with a member of the opposite sex, there is a real emergency in life which must be faced. If you are alone, the dream signifies that there are increased responsibilities either at home or at work which must be faced.

Housewife

A woman who dreams of being a housewife isn't destined for a life of washing dishes and doing chores; rather, she may be with a man who is constantly on the move, for example a salesman, sportsman or actor. The dream expresses no warning about such a relationship, merely indicating that it is the dreamer's chosen path.

Hunting

Any dream of hunting for game is a warning of impending physical danger. If you are hunting for something you have lost, you may rightly fear being bad-mouthed by someone you took to be a friend.

Hypnotism

Being hypnotised in a dream and made to do something against your will means you are hiding a secret which you fear you may be called to account for. This dream warns you to bring the problem into the open on your own terms. If you dream of hypnotising someone else, you may have difficulty meeting debts.

I

Ice
Sitting on ice indicates comfort and happiness with life. Slipping on ice suggests you are planning or will plan a holiday — somewhere warm! Skating alone means you are due some sort of award. Skating with a partner warns that your public behaviour is becoming unreasonable.

Ice-cream
Eating ice-cream in a dream foretells a happy experience, involving children, to come.

Illness
If you dream of being ill, be prepared for a damaging dispute with a lover. If you dream of someone else being ill, you are distressed or worried in life and need to face the source of your upset head-on.

Immorality
Any dream of immorality is not a warning about your own behaviour. Instead it is a warning to you not to judge others too harshly or be unduly suspicious.

Incest
This dream is a warning. Whatever form it takes, the message is that you must not lower your standards — especially moral standards — in life.

Indian
Native North and South Americans are, if friendly in a dream, omens of good luck. If they are hostile, your fears

about a business partner may indeed be well founded.

Inheritance
One of the rare life-mirror dreams. If you dream of being the recipient of a bequest, that is precisely what is likely to happen to you in the near future.

Insanity
Dreaming of a mad person means you are facing a hostile time from a relative who seems, in your view, to be unable to see reason. If you dream that you are insane, fear not; the omen in this dream is of good news to come.

Invention
You don't necessarily have to dream of being a boffin; any dream in which you see yourself working on a new invention means you are close to achieving a lifelong goal.

Invitiation
Dreams of receiving invitations denote additional expenses in life which you really wish you didn't have to incur.

Iron
Dreams of iron tend to indicate a slow, steady progress towards your main objectives in life.

Ironing
For a woman to dream of ironing clothes, the omen is the reverse of the drudgery this chore entails in life; it means she is working towards being relieved of a burden. If a man has this dream, it is a good money omen, possibly indicating an increase in salary.

Island

Your desert island fantasy can come true. If you dream of being alone on an island with a member of the opposite sex you are on the brink of embarking on a wild and adventurous romance.

Itch

Unimportant but nagging worries are indicated by a dream in which you have an itch on any part of your body.

Ivy

Faithfulness in love — both your own and your partner's — is indicated by a dream of ivy growing on a wall or building. If, however, you dream of tearing the ivy down, be warned that you are capable of being unfaithful by drifting into a dangerous liaison. Planting ivy is a sign of wanting to put down roots and establish your current relationship on a permanent basis.

J

Jaguar
To dream of this tiger-like creature of the South American jungle forewarns either a man or a woman of a catty person with a vicious tongue who may be determined to wreck a rival's relationship.

Jail
If you dream of going to jail, you are worried about being caught telling a white lie. To see prisoners being committed to jail means you may be about to suffer illness.

Jar
A single jar or row of jars on a shelf means you will find great pleasure in a new pursuit.

Javelin
Broken relationships or friendships are signalled by a dream in which a javelin is thrown at a person. If it is thrown on an athletics field, purely for sport, then business prospects are good.

Jealousy
Dreams of being jealous of members of the opposite sex — especially a partner — spell gloom and despondency for the dreamer. This is a negative dream with a deep-rooted real-life problem which must be solved.

Jewellery
Wearing jewellery signifies social achievement in your community but dreaming of buying it signifies that you

are trying to cover up a mistake.

Jigsaw
Uncertain love partners who dream of doing a jigsaw puzzle face the break-up of their relationship.

Jilt
If you jilt your lover in a dream you are destined to fail to keep an important appointment. If you are the jilted one, expect luck in money matters.

Joke
If you dream of hearing a joke and laughing heartily at it, then you await an unwelcome visitor. If you are the teller of the joke and your audience laughs, you can afford to be starry-eyed in a current business venture. If no one laughs, be prepared for failure.

Judge
Men who dream of appearing before a judge in court may face an embarrassing grilling from their lovers, who may not believe an explanation about an absence from home.

Juice
Dream of drinking fruit juice and you can expect financial assistance in paying a bill that has been worrying you.

Jumping
This is a fortunate dream, for if you dream of jumping over any sort of obstacle, you find – and will continue to find – all of life's problems easy to solve.

Junk

A pile of junk in your dream means you face confusion and difficulty overcoming a problem which is about to confront you.

K

Kaleidoscope
The myriad colours and shapes of a kaleidoscope in your dream signify that you are keen to buy, or possibly make, new clothes for yourself.

Kangaroo
Dreaming of this Australian creature means you should be ready for a long journey, almost certainly by plane.

Ketchup
Pouring tomato ketchup on your food is a sign that you will continue to feel frustrated by attempts to get to know a good-looking and intriguing new person in your life.

Kettle
Dreams of a boiling kettle mean a happy and contented family life. If the kettle boils dry, though, yours will be a life of woe.

Key/Keyhole
Dreaming of having a key in your hand signifies a current, mild flirtation. If you put the key in a lock, be prepared for your advances to be spurned. Peeping through a keyhole foretells feelings of shame.

Kidnap
If you are kidnapped in a dream, your chosen partner in life is likely to be quite wealthy. But beware, for he or she is unlikely to bring you any lasting happiness.

Killing

If you are the terrified witness to a murder in your dream, you will move to a new home but regret doing so. If you are the killer, either by design or accident, the dream is rebuking you for recent bad manners towards someone.

Kiss

Dreams of kissing occur very frequently and have several interpretations. A married couple kissing signifies contentment; an unmarried couple, happiness now and to come. A woman who dreams of kissing a very old man faces disappointment in life and love. To dream of kissing a baby, after the style of a canvassing politician, indicates success in a difficult task.

Kite

Flying a kite in your dream means you may be biting off more than you can chew. You have, perhaps, taken on a job which is beyond your capabilities. If the kite string breaks, the omen is of bad luck in business.

Kitten

If a woman dreams of a playful young kitten, the current man in her life is likely to be more interested in a brief affair than a lasting love-match.

A man who has a similar dream should treat it as a warning that the woman in his life is simply toying with his affections.

Knapsack

A full knapsack in a dream denotes a pleasant journeyin the near future, whereas an empty one means a rocky financial road ahead.

Knave

Holding any one of the four knaves from a pack of cards means you are about to be tricked into doing something you normally wouldn't even consider.

Knee

If your knees tremble in a dream, it means you should go down on them — to repent a recent sin.

If a man dreams of dimpled knees, he is having, or about to have, an affair with a foreign woman.

Knife

An open knife is a sign of strife, a closed one indicates someone could be out to swindle you. A very dull knife suggests you are struggling to make ends meet financially.

Knitting

To knit in a dream is a most welcome family omen, signifying that you will have healthy children and grandchildren who will adore you.

Knock

If you hear a knock in your dream, be prepared for an exciting encounter — possibly sexual — with a foreigner.

L

Laboratory
You are on the brink of solving a long-standing mystery if you dream of working in a lab.

Lace
Women who dream of lace will be adored for their femininity by many men. Men who dream of women wearing lace underwear can expect a tantalising relationship which may or may not last.

Ladder
If you dream of climbing a ladder and a rung breaks you need never again worry about financial security. If a ladder falls on you, beware malicious gossip. If you dream of having to climb a ladder to get into a house via an upstairs window, you are concerned, or about to be, by a message from someone close.

Lagoon
Boating alone on a quiet lagoon is a portent of danger, possibly on a road. If you are accompanied on the boat, you will soon meet an old friend in exceptional circumstances.

Lake
Dreaming of a stormy lake means that disaster could be heading your way, but if you meet it with grim determination you will be able to turn it into triumph. If you are sailing on a lake and your boat capsizes, family troubles are on the horizon. Sailing in peaceful weather augurs well for peace in life, while sailing by moonlight means a happy

and romantic love affair.

Lane
Young lovers who dream of meeting in a shady, leafy lane will be truly lucky in love — as long as they are discreet about their romance.

Laughter
If you dream of laughing out loud, nothing but good can come your way. To make someone else laugh indicates profitable investments.

Library
Others will applaud your cleverness if you dream of going to a library, especially if your daytime job is of an artistic nature.

Lifeboat
Seeing a lifeboat being launched in a dream means you are about to embark on a new love affair or fresh business venture. If the lifeboat is steady, you will succeed in either. If it capsizes, the reverse is true.

Light
Light in a dream is always more favourable than darkness. Turning on an electric light means a lively party is in the offing. Lighting a candle means a happy meeting is in prospect.

Lightning
Especially if accompanied by torrential rain and thunder in a dream, lightning foretells disaster.

Lingerie

Women who dream of lingerie are almost always gifted social climbers. Black lingerie, however, signifies that your companion loves excitement and is perhaps even more adventurous than you. Men who dream of lingerie should guard against saying the wrong things at the wrong times to women and ruining relationships before they have a chance to blossom (*see also* Lace).

Lion

Workmates and colleagues look up to you and will continue to do so if you dream of a lion. If the lion attacks you and you overcome it, you will acquire even greater leadership qualities.

Lizard

Dreaming about this reptile means you may have slipped up and are about to be exposed for some misdemeanour.

Luck

To dream of being lucky is a sure sign that you will be lucky, yet it is also a gentle warning against taking life too easily.

Lust

Succumbing to wanton lust in a dream may feel sexually exciting but it's a bad omen for your present relationship, signifying that it is based on little or no trust.

M

Machinery
If you dream of clean machines churning out products in a busy workplace, you enjoy an excellent relationship with your employer. If, however, the machines are rusty or standing idle, then your working relationship with your boss is disintegrating fast.

Magnifying glass
Viewing anything under a magnifying glass means that you have, or soon will have, more money to spend than ever.

Maltese cat
Stroking a Maltese cat and hearing it purr contentedly in a dream means a member of the opposite sex with loose morals wants to get his or her claws into you.

Mansion
To dream of living in a mansion does not indicate an imminent windfall that will set you up in style for life. It does, however, suggest extensive travel around the world with your partner.

Marbles
Returning to the childhood pursuit of playing marbles means that a former lover is still hot for you.

Marriage
Dreams of a contented and happy marriage signal quite the opposite in a relationship. They mean you are likely to quarrel with or even split from a current lover.

If a woman dreams of being a bridesmaid at a wedding, it means she is destined for a whirlwind courtship and will be wed soon herself.

If you dream of people crying at a wedding, then divorce is imminent in real life.

Match

A dream in which you strike a match should be treated as — the perfect matchmaker. It means you have already found or will find a love which will prove strong enough to ensure lasting happiness for you and your partner.

Mattress

If you dream of lying on a soft mattress and luxuriating in its comfort, beware your behaviour towards your lover. This dream is a warning that things might not appear to be a comfortable as they appear.

Meadow

Lush pastures in a dream signify that you are enjoying a time of plenty in life. If there is a stream running through the meadow, your fortunes will be even further enhanced.

Medusa

Dreams of the mythical she-beast whose locks of hair turned into poisonous snakes signal extreme danger in a love affair. One you think adores you may, in fact, be scheming against you. If you have this dream, treat every-one of the opposite sex with caution.

Mermaid

This dream will never result in the fantastic romance you may have hoped for. Sadly, it predicts that you are destined to suffer a deep disappointment.

Meteor
Dreaming of a meteor flashing across the sky means that
any success you enjoy will be short-lived.

Microscope
Viewing any object under a microscope in your dream suggests that you are surprised by the behaviour of someone
you were convinced you knew well.

Midget
If you dream of meeting a midget, in life you will meet a
man connected with books or pictures who will become a
close friend.

Milk
Images of milk are among the luckiest of all dream symbols, foretelling a lasting marriage and a peaceful settled
home life. To drink cows' milk augurs well for your health;
goats' milk, for prosperity in business. If you dream of
milking a cow, your future holds comfort and security
through continued hard work.

Miracle
If you witness any form of miracle in your dream, you are
brimful of confidence and your future has never seemed
so secure.

Mirror
If you dream of seeing yourself in a mirror on the wall (or
indeed mounted anywhere) then, just as the saying goes,
you will be deemed the fairest one of all by an ardent

admirer who is waiting to show you true love. But if you break a mirror in your dream, your current love affair is doomed to failure.

Monk/Monastery

To dream of talking to a monk means you have peace of mind and are assured of an easier life in future. If a man dreams of being in a monastery, it's a sign of plain sailing in all aspects of his life. If, however, a woman has this dream, she will be accused of — and is more likely to be guilty of — some form of deception, possibly in love.

Moon

To dream of seeing a full moon, especially if it is reflected in water, means huge success in your love-life. A clear, silvery moon in a cloudless sky denotes success in a new pursuit. Looking at the moon over your left shoulder prophesies a month of good luck. But if your vision of the moon becomes obscured by clouds, brace yourself for a number of setbacks.

Moth

Malicious lies will be spread about you if you dream of trying to catch a moth. If, in your dream, you succeed in catching and killing it, you will vanquish your enemies and detractors. If you dream of clothing riddled with moths or moth-holes, then your immediate family will face sadness.

Mountain

Climbing a mountain in your dream foretells promotion at work. Scaling a steep mountain with an icy peak means you will overcome seemingly insurmountable obstacles to achieve your goal.

Mouth
Dreaming of a beautiful mouth means your love-life will reach new heights of ecstasy. If you see the mouth of a baby, a person you know only vaguely will turn out to be a good and trusted friend. Seeing a cruel mouth in your dreams cautions you against being too quick to criticise others. If the teeth are bared, you face being hurt by someone you trusted or even loved.

Mushroom
To dream of picking or eating mushrooms means that through taking intelligent risks you are capable of acquiring a great deal of money.

Music
Hearing music in a dream is an omen of good luck, as long as the music is in tune. If it is discordant you will have reason to rue a decision or feel discouraged about a current project.

Mustard
Dream of eating mustard and the chances are you're hot stuff. If mustard does figure in your dream get set for a sexual relationship that you've longed for to take off in a big way.

N

Nail
To dream of hammering in a nail means you are destined to accomplish a task you thought was way beyond your power or ability.

Napkin
Using a napkin to wipe your mouth or hands in a dream means you will satisfactorily complete a new task which has been assigned to you. If you dream of folding a napkin, expect an invitation to the home of someone you have been hoping to visit for some time.

Napoleon
If you dream of seeing Napoleon Bonaparte, your current restlessness in life is likely to continue for some time. If you dream of being Napoleon, don't worry — you haven't gone mad. This dream is simply warning you that you are about to attract criticism, possibly from someone close.

Nausea
Feeling sick in a dream means you are about to fall under suspicion or be accused of something you did not do.

Navy
If you dream of being in the navy, your sex life will be plain sailing and you will attract many admirers.

Neck
A pain in your neck in a dream means that someone in life you don't like is gunning for you and could cause trouble.

If you dream of a voluptuous woman's neck, you are climbing the social ladder. But if the neck is thin and scrawny, you are about to lose money.

Necklace
A woman who dreams of wearing a necklace is falling for, or will fall for, a distinguished man with whom she will spend a great deal of time. A man who dreams of giving his girlfriend or wife a necklace as a gift will soon enjoy good luck.

Neon light
Dreaming of a neon light means you have already become bored with someone new in your life.

Nettle
If you dream of being stung by a nettle, it means you must assert yourself in life. This dream implores you to stand up for your rights.

Newspaper
If you dream of buying a newspaper, a surprise — perhaps not a pleasant one — is in store.

Nipple
Any adult who dreams of suckling at a nipple is, in fact, worried about personal debts.

Noodles
A dream in which you eat noodles suggests you are unhappy with where you are living and would perhaps welcome a move to a quieter location.

Nose

A man who dreams of touching or tweaking a woman's nose is, perhaps only subconsciously, preparing to wed and will more than likely be married within a year of the dream.

If a woman dreams of kissing a man on the nose, trouble with a relative is on her horizon.

Blowing your nose in a dream predicts that you are on the verge of shaking off debts.

Nougat

A dream in which you eat nougat suggests you have become or are about to become part of a group of exotic people with whom you may spend a great deal of time but will never come truly to like or trust.

Nudity/Nakedness

Sheer bliss awaits lovers who dream of nudity if, in the dream, the beauty of the human body is admired. But if any lecherous thoughts or feelings invade the dream, be prepared for a period of discontent with your loved one. To dream of being naked in a crowd of people means you feel guilty — and fear being found out — about a minor deception.

Nun

To dream of seeing or talking to a nun means you feel more settled and at ease with life than you did previously.

Nurse

To dream of a nurse in her trim uniform is a portent of a new source of income. If a man dreams of falling in love with a nurse, he is set for a lucky break at work.

Nut

Cracking a nut in your dream signifies success in a major project you are currently working on. Eating a nut suggests you will succumb to some form of temptation unless you are totally resolute.

Nymph

Dreaming of a nymph is a sign of a strange but exhilarating outdoor experience in store.

O

Oak
To dream of oak trees means you are assured peace of mind and a comfortable income.

Oar
To dream of breaking an oar while rowing indicates that you are destined for trouble which, if you use your brain, you will eventually overcome.

Oasis
A dream in which you arrive at an oasis after a long, hot journey predicts considerable success in a new venture.

Occult/Ouija board
A dream in which you attend a spiritualist meeting or are involved in any way with investigators of the occult warns that friends are likely to be critical of your oversensitivity.

Ocean
An ocean cruise in your dream means you want to — and almost certainly will — escape from someone who has been causing you trouble. To swim in the ocean means you must take time to relax away from daily worries.

To see an ocean with calm water predicts money luck. If the ocean is choppy, with crashing waves, the reverse is true and bad luck in business lies ahead.

Ointment
Any dream in which ointment is rubbed into your or someone else's body suggests that you may be pursuing

someone of the opposite sex who will not turn out to be an ideal partner for you.

Opera
A dream in which you go to the opera foretells that you will be tempted to deceive someone close, possibly even your lover.

Organ
If, in your dream, you hear the strains of organ music, rest assured that you partner is deeply in love with you. If you dream of playing the organ, expect soon to be asked to be a bridesmaid or best man at a wedding.

Orgy
Dreaming of taking part in an orgy — especially a drunken orgy — is a sign that you must be more careful about the company you keep. You could fall foul of the law unless you take great care after this dream.

Owl
An owl is a dream omen of evil but if you manage to scare or drive away an owl in your dream, your circumstances are set to improve. Dreaming of an owl flying into your home predicts a visit to feuding relatives.

P

Paint
If you dream of painting anything, you have something to hide from your partner. To dream of seeing a house being painted means someone is keeping a secret from you.

Parrot
A group of noisy, squawking parrots in a dream means you will have to attend a gathering of mainly women.

To dream of teaching a caged parrot obscene words means you will have to defend your name.

Parsnip
Dream parsnips portend broken friendships. They also warn you not to be too easily satisfied.

Petal
Pulling petals from a flower is a dream sign that an engagement or long-standing relationship is about to come to an end.

Pheasant
To hunt or shoot pheasants in a dream indicates that although your short-term future may be financially secure, you are well advised to save for a rainy day. To dream of eating pheasant means you can expect income from a new source.

Pigeon
If you dream of pigeons flying in a circle above you, be prepared for family disharmony. Feeding these birds is a

sign that you are too easily distracted in life.

Pirate
Dreaming of old-time pirates like Long John Silver predicts a car accident. This dream urges great caution.

Polar bear
Seeing a polar bear in a zoo predicts misery through the loss of treasured possessions. If, however, you see a polar bear in its natural icy environment, your family fortunes are set to improve.

Police
It is always a good luck omen to dream of policemen — unless you happen to be on the run from them. Dreaming of being stopped by a traffic cop means you will have to apologise to a friend for letting him or her down.

Poodle
You are set for amusing experiences if you dream of a poodle, especially if its fur has been clipped to look trendy.

Porthole
To dream of looking through a ship's porthole and seeing another vessel on the horizon means you are set for an exciting adventure with someone — possibly a future partner — you haven't seen for years.

Portrait
Dreaming of having your portrait drawn or painted, or of being photographed, means you are deeply disillusioned about someone or something in life. Watching someone else having his or her portrait executed means you can

expect to be invited to a select social gathering.

Poverty
Dreams of poverty are only bad luck if they are accompanied by dirt or degradation. Otherwise, they actually predict an upswing of your fortunes.

Priest
Whatever denomination the priest may be, this dream is always a good luck omen.

Pulpit
You may be about to be suspected or accused of double-dealing if you dream of delivering a sermon from a pulpit.

Q

Quarantine
Dreaming of being held in quarantine signals great unhappiness — unless in the dream you show a clean bill of health which results in your release.

Quarrel
Dreaming of quarrelling with your lover actually predicts early marriage. A man who dreams of arguing with a strange woman will come off second best in a dispute with his boss at work. A dream of quarrelling with a neighbour portends travel by bus. A family quarrel in a dream suggests you may move home.

Quarry
If you dream of working in a quarry, hewing out chunks of rock, you are destined to work hard throughout your life but never for great reward.

Quay
You are destined for a foreign holiday if you dream of ships berthed at a quay.

Queen
A woman who dreams of being a queen afforded great reverence by her subjects, is in fact in danger of being hotly pursued by creditors.

To dream of kneeling before a queen prophesies promotion at work. If, however, you dream of kissing the queen's hand, you are in danger of falling victim to office or workplace politics.

Seeing a queen pass by in a grand carriage signifies happiness and prosperity.

Quicksand
A nightmare in which you slowly sink into quicksand should be treated as a warning against prying into the affairs of other people. If you dream of rescuing someone from quicksand your financial affairs are well-starred.

Quiz
If you dream of answering questions in a quiz the omen is good if you get the answers right. But be prepared for bad luck if you don't.

R

Rabbi

If you are Jewish and dream of seeking advice from a rabbi, you will be lucky in business. If you are of any other religious denomination, you will meet a new friend who will help you enormously.

Rabbit

Seeing many rabbits in a dream signifies that you will have several children, all of whom will be a credit to you. To go hunting rabbits prophesies that while travelling you will meet someone of the opposite sex who interests you.

Rabies

If you dream of being attacked by a mad dog or any salivating, enraged wild animal, beware of enemies plotting behind your back.

Race

Lovers who dream of any kind of race — on foot, on horseback, by car, or any other such form of contest — are sure of happy and prosperous married life, should they choose to get wed. If you dream of running a foot race, whether you win or lose you are likely to be offered a new position at work. To dream of hating taking part in a race is an omen of bad luck.

Radio

If you dream of hearing a radio playing quietly in the background, look forward to peaceful days spent in the company of your family. If the radio is loud, blaring or irritating, the dream foretells a rheumatism or arthritis attack.

Raft
If you dream of slowly floating down a river on a raft, you should be warned against indolence, which may be slowing you down in life. But if the river is fast-flowing, your progress in life in any direction you choose will be swift.

Rage
If you dream of flying into a rage yourself, be prepared to be snubbed by someone you would really like to impress.

To dream of trying to pacify someone else who is in a rage augurs bad luck in any project in which you are currently involved.

Rain
Torrential rain which soaks you to the skin is a rotten dream omen for lovers; it predicts a cold reception from your partner.

To watch rain from indoors suggests you are about to suffer deep disappointment in business.

Rainbow
As in life, you may find yourself chasing a dream rainbow for that elusive pot of gold. Just as in life, it can be a frustrating quest, but if you finally overcome all the troubles and obstacles in your way and reach the end of the rainbow, greater happiness than you have ever known before is in prospect.

Raisin
A dream about raisins, either seeing them or eating them, signifies that your strength of character is building, and

will see you through future problems in life.

Rake
If you dream of using a rake in the garden, you are about to have an enjoyable time with your family. To dream of stepping on a rake accidentally, so that its handle flies up and hits you, should prepare you for a surprise; however, unlike in your dream, it will be a pleasant one.

Rape
Any dream which involves rape is a stark warning to steer clear of evil or any kind of misdeed.

Rat
Serious illness is forecast by the dream vision of a rat. This dream warns you to avoid crowds and take care of your health.

Razor
A man who dreams of shaving with an old-fashioned, cut-throat razor is likely to meet and fall for an old-fashioned girl with a strict moral code. If a man dreams of shaving with a modern safety razor he is in line for plaudits from his employer. If he dreams of cutting himself with a razor he can expect to answer for bad actions he had not expected to be discovered. To dream of fighting or slashing someone with a razor signifies years of abject poverty.

Reading
If you dream of reading aloud from a book, newspaper or magazine, you are destined to meet someone rich who will be of great help in your life. Reading, not necessarily aloud, is always a good omen in a dream; in particular,

reading books predicts a settled home life.

Red
If you dream in colour and red is the predominant colour, you are set for major disturbances in your life.

Redhead
If a man dreams of a red-haired woman he is liable to be caught out by his indiscretions. If a woman dreams of a redheaded man, she should prime herself for an argument with her lover or husband.

Reindeer
Dreaming, not necessarily of fictitious Rudolph, but of any reindeer, whether it is roaming free or hitched to a sleigh, does not mean you're looking forward to Christmas or have preoccupations about it. Instead, it signals the fact that a possession you considered to be worthless will prove to be just the opposite.

Retirement
Dreams of retiring from work do not mean that you are, in reality, nearing the end of your working life. They mean you are due to get a pay rise, though the volume of work you will be expected to complete will increase commensuratel or even disproportionately.

Revenge
Any dream in which you exact revenge against an enemy or rival is a bad sign, especially for females. It augurs bad luck and possibly illness.

Rhinoceros

If rhino horn is a purported aphrodisiac, then dreaming of the beast itself in a zoo might be expected to provide a tremendous boost to a would-be lover. Indeed it is a strong indicator that members of the opposite sex will pursue you vigorously. If, however, you dream of a rhino in the wild, be prepared to be inundated with bills.

Ride

Riding in any kind of vehicle signifies that you are about to receive news of a distant relative.

Riot

Try to curb a lifestyle in which you crave the sensual and luxurious for you and your lover. This dream strongly warns against being too free and easy — especially in your spending — with members of the opposite sex.

River

Dreams of sitting on a river bank, idly watching boats, waterfowl or just the water pass by, is a sure sign that you are heading in the right direction in life and will thoughtfully overcome any problem or impediment.

Robbery

If you dream that a robbery is committed in your home and something you deeply treasure is stolen, prepare to receive a present which gives you immense pleasure. If you dream of a robber tying you up, get ready for great entertainment!

Rope

Handling rope in a dream is a sign that you will meet a

new friend for whom you are willing to make sacrifices.

Rosary
Counting the beads of a rosary, whether you are Catholic or not, is heralds great peace of mind and an improvement in your living conditions.

Rose
Dreaming of a rose of any colour signifies deep love. Rose dreams are wonderful for those with new partners, predicting lasting joy. Faded roses imply the impending loss of a close friend. Artificial roses mean someone you trust implicitly is about to deceive you.

Rubber
Dreaming of rubber in any shape or form predicts good health and freedom from worry.

Ruby
If a woman dreams of wearing a ruby, she will be chased by many ardent admirers.

S

Sabotage
Being involved in sabotage or wilfully wrecking something in a dream predicts a terrible collision in life with someone with whom you are closely involved.

Saddle
If you dream that, while riding a horse, you feel the saddle slipping, take heed that you are not paying enough attention to your work.

Salt
Dreaming of sprinkling salt on food does, perversely, mean that you may be about to suffer from food poisoning.

Sand
Dreaming of sand indicates irritation with someone you feel may be using you to further their own prospects.

Sausage
Let's be clear that the sausage is not a phallic symbol. However, if you dream of eating sausages, there is indeed a sexual connotation, which is that you feel guilty of — or may be accused of — stealing someone's partner.

Saxophone
If you dream of hearing a saxophone, expect an invitation to a wild party where the booze will flow and inhibitions will be thrown aside. If you dream of playing it, expect a row with someone close, probably of the opposite sex.

Scaffold

If you dream of scaffolding surrounding a building, new opportunities at work will arise. If you dream of a hangman's scaffold, however, something dreadful is due to happen close to home.

Scales

Weighing food on kitchen scales indicates you will always have plenty to eat. Weighing yourself on bathroom scales or stand-on scales in public presages disappointment or worry. If you dream of scraping the scales off a fish, there may be a plot afoot aimed at discrediting you.

Scandal

A dream in which you are ensnared in a scandal, public or private, suggests you should clear your conscience of something that has been bothering you. If you dream of causing a scandal for someone else, you are likely to be accused of dishonesty.

School

If you dream of going back to your old school or dream of when you were at school, look forward to a happy encounter with an old friend.

Scissors

Cutting anything with a pair of scissors in a dream suggests you will be the victim of a friend or workmate's humorous prank. Dreaming of using scissors with your left hand predicts an interesting discovery.

Seagull

If you dream of seeing seagulls flying, you're on the brink

of an adventure. It will, however, be one of a largely innocent nature.

Sex
Dreaming about sex, the principal subject of this book, actually means virtually nothing at all. There are very few dreams which, at some stage, do not involve sex. They are certainly not normally wish-fulfilment dreams. If, however, you dream of sex in purely functional, biological terms, it portends a long and happy life.

Singing
If you dream of singing before an audience you are not a flamboyant person, but crave solitude. You should consider spending more time alone. To be part of a choir, congregation or group where you join in with the chorus suggests good companionship and the friendship of many.

Skeleton
If you dream of discovering a human skeleton you are likely to face ridicule over fears you harbour but which others feel are unfounded.

Skirt
If a woman dreams that her skirt is too short or too long, she feels troubled about things which should really be disregarded.

A man who dreams of a leggy woman wearing a short skirt should take great heart; he is set to enjoy good luck in all aspects of his life.

Sky
The blazing colours of sunset or sunrise in a dream predict

a helter-skelter love-life which will, sadly, end in despair. Grey skies, though, suggest a dear friend will stick by you through thick and thin.

Smoke

If you dream of seeing or smelling smoke in a dream without being aware of its source, you face a period of worry and concern. However, to see smoke coming from a fire or chimney is a sign of an increase in income.

Soap

Sweet-smelling scented soap in a dream suggests moonlight and roses with the partner who is precious in your life. Soap that smells of antiseptic suggests that you are ill at ease in company.

Son

A person who dreams of his or her real-life son is certain to achieve happiness.

Sparrow

Dreaming about this common bird indicates, sadly, a never-ending struggle to make ends meet.

Spire

Any dream in which you see a church spire means you will be blessed throughout life by friendship and love. If, however, the spire leans to one side slightly, you may face difficulties achieving your ambitions.

Spirit

Dreaming of summoning spirits or receiving messages from beyond the grave through a ouija board means that someone, perhaps your lover, will betray you by revealing to others a secret you share.

Squirrel
If you feed a squirrel in your dream you're set for good times with close friends. A squirrel in a cage, forlornly treading in circles on a revolving wheel, foretells a hopeless love life.

Stadium
To dream of being at a stadium for an event like a football match or pop concert means a round of parties and social events will go with a swing — and you'll be one of the liveliest guests.

Stairs
To dream of falling down stairs means someone is trying to lure you into a conspiracy which should be avoided at all costs. If you dream of falling up stairs and are unmarried, you are destined for peace of mind. But if you are married, be prepared for a brief unsettled period. To sweep or scrub stairs in a dream suggests an improvement in living conditions.

Star
A bright, beaming star in the sky signifies that a member of the opposite sex will help you realise a long-standing ambition.

Starvation
Dreaming of being starved is a terrible bad luck omen. It should be taken as a warning to save as much money as you can now to stave off poor financial fortunes in the near

future. Dreaming of seeing others starving means you will suffer many unhappy days.

Stealing
Dreams of stealing caution against new deals or investments. A dream of being caught, ironically, is a good omen

Strike
If you dream of going on strike, the exact opposite will befall you at work. You'll make tremendous progress and please your boss.

String
A dream of saving or putting aside string you have untied from packages or parcels means others will laugh at you for being over-fussy or prim.

Striptease
Be warned to behave if you dream of seeing a sexy woman strip. For men only, this dream predicts disgrace unless you clean up your lifestyle immediately.

Submarine
Being on a submarine in a dream means you will have to explain you absence from a function you were expected to attend. If you dream of firing a torpedo from a submarine, an incident involving a member of the opposite sex will have a profound effect on your life.

Suffocation
If you have a nightmare of being suffocated, be careful to avoid large gatherings of people and try to stay in the open air as much as possible.

Suitcase

Packing a suitcase does not mean you are about to embark on a long journey or holiday as you might expect. Instead, it means you are about to be visited by someone you find tiresome who may long overstay their welcome.

Sunflower

Dreaming of sunflowers means you are in danger of making a public spectacle of yourself unless you are exceptionally careful. Eating sunflower seeds means you are likely to encounter an old friend when you least expect it.

Swan

Graceful white swans in a dream predict a happy married life. Flying swans portend healthy children and an equally healthy income.

Sword

Any dream of a sword fight indicates that someone you are at loggerheads with in life should, instead, be treated as a friend and ally. To dream of wearing a sword means you are destined for a higher position, either at work or socially.

T

Table

Different types of table convey vastly different dream messages. If you dream of sitting at a card table, a new opportunity to make money will arise. If it is a kitchen table, hard work for a small salary is indicated. A dining-room table suggests happy social times ahead. A library or home-study table denotes promotion at work.

Tail

If, in a bizarre dream, you imagine you have a tail, you are likely to feel obliged to apologise for the actions of some-one else, possibly a relative.

Dreaming of pulling the tail of a dog or cat is an omen of impending sickness.

Tattoo

Being tattoed in a dream signals travel by land or sea. Seeing someone in a dream with strange designs on his or her body indicates that you will be told a story which must not be repeated.

Teacher

If you dream of meeting a former schoolteacher of yours, you can expect to be called upon to make a donation to charity. If you dream of being a teacher, get set for headaches, both physical and mental.

Telephone

The sound of a telephone ringing in a dream foretells trouble or illness. If you dream of making a phone call, you will meet an old friend you may not have seen for many years. If you dream of trying to use a phone which doesn't work, anticipate the illness of a loved one.

Television
Watching television in your dream generally augurs well for increased business profits.

Theatre
If you dream of being in a theatre during the performance of a play, expect many happy hours with friends. But if the theatre is dark and empty, a period of intense boredom will be your lot.

Thunder
Rolling, growling thunder in a dream warns you to beware of treachery by acquaintances whom you may have long suspected of double-dealing and conniving. However, if you hear thunder cracking, you may be on the way towards solving a long-term problem in life.

Tidal wave
Dreams of a devastating tidal wave predict death in the family, or the death of someone close.

Tiger
Being attacked by a dream tiger is a portent of a family dispute which will have far-reaching repercussions. Killing or driving away a tiger in a dream means that there will perhaps still be a dispute but you will be the peacemaker who settles it.

Tomato
Eating fresh or tinned tomatoes in a dream suggests extensive travel which will bring you great enjoyment. Drinking tomato juice heralds travel by air.

Towel
Dreaming of drying your face or hands on a cloth towel augurs prosperity and good health. If the towel is made of paper, though, the reverse is true. If you find a soggy towel, be prepared for disquieting news. If you dream of hitting someone with a wet towel you are in danger of losing your position at work.

Traffic
To dream of watching traffic on a busy road means a new and vexing problem is about to confront you at work. Being stuck in a traffic jam predicts serious difficulties, though sailing through traffic means business or family problems will be easily solved.

Train
Dream travel by train urges you to pay closer attention to detail at work and thereby achieve more.

Trapeze
If a woman dreams she is a trapeze artiste in a circus, she can look forward to meeting a handsome, genuine man who will eventually propose marriage. To dream of falling from a trapeze is a warning against making a wrong decision which could have dire consequences.

Treasure
Discovering treasure in a dream is a portent of travel and

excitement which will bring immense pleasure, though not yield any great financial improvement.

Tree
Planting a tree is a brilliant dream symbol for lovers. It signifies a June wedding, a romantic honeymoon and a blissful married life.

To cut down a tree in a dream, however, is an omen of bad luck in love.

Trial
If you dream of facing trial in court, you will in real life face a complex problem which will utterly frustrate you.

Trumpet
Blowing a trumpet in your dream suggests a surprise which will delight you.

Tulip
This is the dream flower for lovers. If you dream of brightly coloured tulips, pucker your lips in waiting for a kiss which will herald a new and exciting love affair. Planting tulip bulbs, however, foretells disappointment.

Tunnel
A dream in which you find yourself travelling through a dark tunnel predicts great difficulty, after which you will finally achieve your heart's desire.

Turkey
Killing a turkey is a good luck omen. Dressing one is an omen of plenty. Seeing a flock of turkeys means you will soon attend a number of public meetings.

Typewriter

If you dream of using a typewriter you should be ready for advancement, most probably at work. If the keys stick or the ribbon jams, however, unsettling news is due to reach you. Strangely, it's bad luck to dream of writing love letters on a typewriter.

U

Umbrella

Dreams of opening and sheltering under an umbrella in a downpour mean you will soon face setbacks in life.

To dream of carrying an unfurled umbrella when the sun is shining means you will receive startling news which will have a radical effect on your plans for the future.

Undertaker

Dreams of a solemn-faced undertaker mean that someone is trying to cheat you out of what is rightfully yours.

Undressing

If you dream of seeing a member of the opposite sex undressing, beware of how far you trust a new person in your life.

Uniform

To dream of wearing any sort of uniform means you are destined to be rewarded for a kind or brave deed.

University

If you dream you are a university student, whetever business or work you are involved in, it is a positive omen showing that life holds a bright future for you.

Urn

A funeral urn which contains someone's ashes predicts travel to unusual yet interesting places. If you dream of flowers in an urn, calm and happiness are yours. However, if the urn is empty or has flowers which have wilted, sad times are in prospect.

V

Vaccination
Painful though a vaccination may be, if you dream of receiving one, expect huge sucess in the work you enjoy the most.

Valentine
If you dream of being sent a prettily decorated Valentine card, you'll soon kiss someone who will turn your head and maybe your heart.

Vampire
If you dream of being attacked by a vampire, be prepared for some unnerving or unsettling experiences. However, if you manage to kill or drive away a vampire you are destined for good luck, especially in affairs of the heart.

Vacuum cleaner
Dreams of doing the hoovering predict great success in joint ventures with a member of the opposite sex.

Velvet
Wearing velvet in a dream means you have done, or are about to do, something you'll be forced to live down later.

If a woman dreams of making a velvet dress, she'll meet a handsome man who will woo her passionately.

Venetian blinds
Act with great caution after a dream in which venetian blinds figure. This dream warns of the dire consequences that will follow an ill-advised act.

Vicar

If you dream of a vicar, expect to be invited to a party dominated by women.

Vinegar

If you dream of tasting vinegar you face being called to account for not being somewhere you should have been.

Violin

If you dream of playing the violin, you face criticism for what others believe to be your strange ideas about life, but on the other hand you will be much admired for your friendliness and generosity.

Virgin

An unmarried woman who dreams of being a virgin will welcome the attentions of many male friends. However, a woman who is married can expect a disturbing episode in her life.

Volcano

An erupting volcano in your dream suggests an altercation with a neighbour that will upset or annoy you but will ultimately prove to be trivial.

W

Watch
Wearing a watch in a dream means that someone of importance is keeping his or her eye on you. Wearing an old-fashioned watch — a fob-watch, for example — means you will be called upon to look after a young person.

Water/Waterfall
Drinking cold water in a dream is a lucky omen. Throwing water at someone suggests you will be unpopular. If you dream of hot water you could well end up in hot water at home or work.

To see a scenic waterfall in a dream means you will meet a good-looking person of the opposite sex who will show you enormous kindness.

Wealth
If you dream of being enormously wealthy you may suffer what at first appears to be a financial upset yet in the end turns out to be something of benefit to you.

Wedding
Dreaming of going to your own wedding means you are destined for happiness in love. If you dream of going to someone else's wedding, be prepared to meet new friends. Eating wedding cake in a dream portends a long life with your current lover.

Weed
Dreams of garden weeds caution you to defend your good name against a scurrilous and unfounded allegation that

someone is making against you.

Whale
If you dream of whales, expect an encouraging improvement in your relationships with acquaintances.

Wheel
Dreams of rotating wheels foretell hard work in prospect, though good results from your endeavours. If a wheel comes off your car while it is in motion, adventure lies ahead. An old wheel at the side of the road predicts disappointment.

Wheelbarrow
Pushing a loaded wheelbarrow in a dream heralds wonderful companionship with someone of the opposite sex. Seeing a wheelbarrow upside down predicts that you will have to bear a heavy burden in life.

Whip
To dream of whipping an animal means someone is set to derive pleasure from making you squirm.

Window
Opening a window in a dream foretells better health. Closing one means you can expect a visitor. Entering a house through a window means someone is speaking ill of you. Breaking a pane of glass indicates a period of poor health.

Wishbone
Breaking a wishbone and making a wish with a member of the opposite sex indicates that you are about to

receive a sizeable legacy.

Witch
Dreams of witches on broomsticks foretell good times ahead with friends.

Wolf
To be chased by wolves means you will be forced to borrow money to survive. If you can kill them or chase them off, your financial problems will be temporary.

X

X-rays

If you dream of having X-rays taken of any part of you, something mysterious is due to happen to a close friend. If you dream of seeing your own bones with X-ray vision, you're about to be called to account for an indiscretion.

Y

Yacht
Partying on a dream yacht is a sure sign that your finances are due to perk up. If you dream of being on board a yacht in rough seas and feel seasick, count on good luck at work. Talking to someone of the opposite sex on a yacht foretells a contented love life.

Youth
An older person who dreams of youthful days is assured continuing ease and comfort.

Z

Zebra
You're set to visit friends if you dream of a zebra. If, however, the animal is dead in your dream, someone you know is about to serve a prison sentence.

Zoo
Exotic travel is forecast if you dream of animals in a zoo. If you dream of taking a child to the zoo you are about to have great luck in money matters.

CHAPTER SEVEN

HOW TO HAVE BETTER SEXUAL DREAMS AND HELP YOUR RELATIONSHIP

Earlier I explained that a dream about a sexual encounter, whether it is a chaste kiss or raging sexual passion, is not necessarily a dream about sex. Generally speaking, such dreams reflect our attitude to life and our emotions. Bearing that in mind, it is possible to find answers to problems we are having within our relationships — both with work colleagues and more intimate partners.

More than 40 years ago the American sex researcher Alfred Kinsey found that in a survey 70 per cent of women admitted to having a sex dream at some point in their lives. These covered all aspects of sex but the one thing they had in common was that a great majority of women found sex dreams distressing. They felt dirty and ashamed of their nocturnal naughtiness. Their dreams tended to reflect a sense of frustration — in both their sexual desires and their daily life.

However, some sexual dreams, particularly those of women, have a foundation in a bad sexual experience or in sexual abuse. These distressing dreams are like a graphic flashback to the event. Such dreams we make no attempt to analyse here; sufferers usually need to undergo counselling to come to terms with their past.

But our sexual dreams need not be anything to be ashamed of. They can help us to release into our lives a creativity that can improve our erotic experiences with our partners.

During our waking hours we often deny that we have needs and fears that trouble us, preferring instead to push them to the back of our minds. In contrast, when we dream, that conscious decision is over-ridden and floodgates are opened.

Not surprisingly, our dreams tend to focus on our relationships. In them daytime inhibitions are thrown to one side and we do things that we think are completely at odds with our personalities.

The messages we get from our sexual dreams can help us resolve relationship problems, and they can be divided into four different areas. By applying the lessons we learn from our dreams, we can improve our relationships or find help in deciding if it is time to end a partnership that is going nowhere.

The four areas are: our emotional needs; advice about relationships; fear of intimacy; and sexual hang-ups. When considering your dream, bear in mind what is going on with your life now and the relevance of the subject matter of your dream.

If you want an answer to a specific problem, you can help to trigger your mind to address it while you sleep. Humans are instinctive creatures, but we have lost the art of tuning into our intuition and listening to it. A perfect example is the way we react when we first meet someone. Social graces come to the fore and we make polite chit-chat and appear to interact with each other. However you should trust the way you feel about someone because we not only communicate verbally, but also with our body language, the way we smile, even the way we smell.

First impressions are usually correct and are born out of pure instinct or a 'gut feeling' you get from someone. And in the same way we get a feeling when all is not quite right within our relationships. To stay in a relationship, everybody has to compromise to some degree. Niggly things are shoved to the back in the face of more practical problems, but it's the niggly things that get you in the end — the kind of things to which we are blinded by the blaze of a new passion.

Our dreams are unencumbered with social behaviour or practical things like mortgage repayments, and therefore they are clear channels in which pure answers can be found. These may be as drastic as leaving the man you thought was your perfect partner. Whether you act on the solutions is up to you.

In helping you to find the answers to relationship difficulties, dreams can also show you that something that you avoided doing can in fact be of great pleasure to you. If you have any particular sexual hang-ups then the dream state can help you to overcome them.

A good example is where a female dreamer finds the thought of oral sex disgusting. Her lover, on the other hand, finds it highly erotic. Her hang-up is rooted in her repressive upbringing. Sex was either avoided in conversation, or if did crop up, it seemed to be regarded as a necessary evil for producing children. Therefore from an early age the dreamer failed to associate sex with pleasure.

The dreamer is anxious to please her lover because in all other areas of their lives they are highly compatible. In her dream the penis is replaced by a sweet lollipop which she enjoys sucking. When she wakes this positive image is in her mind and the next time she and her partner make love, she initiates oral sex.

Dreams can also help you to recognise how healthy your relationship is. While we tend to ignore the warning signals evident in daily life, in dreams they scream out at us.

Throughout an ever-changing relationship, dreams remain the one thing that is constant, reflecting the changes but remaining true to ourselves.

When people choose partners, they tend to gravitate towards relationships with people who provide a degree of familiarity. Often they pick partners who are of the same type as an earlier boyfriend. An example would be of a woman whose boyfriends have all liked to dominate her — they might have different personalities in other ways, but share similarly dominant traits — and each time she falls for the same kind of person. Her relationships end in tears every time, but she never sees and acts on the warning signs that predict the end.

By recording your dreams during a relationship, you can use them as a huge warning signal before you get in too deep. And while your heart is singing with passion, your dreams will be bringing you down to earth in a healthy, constructive way.

Being involved in a dead-end relationship is very damaging for self-esteem. But it is very difficult to break patterns that have been set up for years and that you have gone along with for the sake of peace. Even if you can see that the relationship is damaging, fear of starting out on your own again will make you think twice. After all, the devil you know...

Trying to change these patterns may help you to mend your self-esteem. Dreams can help you see through to the core of the problem and provide solutions that your normally troubled mind cannot come up with. Listen to your dreams and act as Fiona did after her dream.

She had been going out with Tom for two years. They first met when her previous relationship, which was very damaging, had just broken up. She had been feeling downtrodden and unloved by a boyfriend who constantly demanded that she share responsibility for their home on an equal basis. She kept to the bargain, but whenever her boyfriend, a photographer, felt like it, he abandoned all responsibility, spending the mortgage money on a piece of photographic equipment he fancied.

So when she met Tom, Fiona couldn't believe it when he took the initiative and made sure that the household ran smoothly. She was happy to take a back seat and allow him to do that and even when he started to organise her day and set out little chores for her to complete, she went along with it. Fiona was just happy that she didn't have to bear all the responsibility for a change.

After a while, however, she felt niggled that everything she wanted to do had to be cleared with Tom. She had quite a disturbing dream in which Tom was going through a list of things for her to do, and when she woke, her overriding feeling was of wanting to break the chains that bound her.

She felt that she ought to be free to make some decisions herself and she thrashed out a deal with Tom telling him that he had to relinquish the control he had imposed on their daily lives. To her surprise, he was very relieved. He was beginning to feel the strain of proving that he was not like her old boyfriend and that he could be relied upon. New ground rules were laid down and the relationship flourished.

In order to use your dream to help you, it is important to address yourself to your worries. Before you go to sleep, follow the procedure described in Chapter 2. I will repeat the checklist for your convenience, but this time with minor changes to reflect the emphasis on solving relationship problems.

1. Jot down in your dream journal some details about the previous day.

2. Put your paper and pen or tape recorder beside your bed, ready for use.

3. Sit on the side of your bed in a relaxed state of mind and tell yourself that you are going to remember your dream when you wake.

4. Concentrate on what you feel is creating a problem for you in your relationship. Ask yourself the question you want answered. For example, 'Is our relationship stable?' or 'Should I stay with him/her?'

5. Record your dreams as soon as you wake up.

6. Note the key symbols.

7. Refer to Chapter 6 to study the general meanings of dream symbols.

8. Apply your findings to your current situation.

In addition, it is important to create a perfect dream scenario by setting the right mood in your bedroom. Consider how much time you spend in the bedroom — you most probably wouldn't dream of having a living room that was not comfortable and that didn't reflect your personality. The reality is that you spend far more time in your bedroom. Just because you tend to sleep through much of that time doesn't mean that you shouldn't care what it looks or feels like.

Of primary concern is the bed. A bad bed equals a bad night. Choose your bed carefully. Test it out before you buy it. Don't be shy, for after all you are the one who has to sleep in it. Get one that gives your body decent support, because back ache wrecks both your sleeping and waking hours.

The colours in your room are important as well. Colour affects our moods, as marketing professionals know and use to advantage. Our bedrooms should be inviting and restful. The colour of the walls, the bed covers, the sheets and even the pillowcases, all affect our moods.

Some deeper shades can be depressing, while vivid colours may bring vitality into your life. Alternatively, some sombre shades can be soothing and womblike, while some bright colours can provoke hyperactivity.

Choose your shades from the appropriate part of the spectrum for the mood you wish to inspire, and decorate your bedroom accordingly – but before choosing a colour make sure it is compatible with your personality. If you are not a pink, gentle and fluffy person, then having a pink bedroom would probably annoy you more than make you feel cosy and comfortable — moods associated with this particular group of colours.

Blue is seen as a spiritual colour, cool, calm and intelligent. Green is a colour associated with vitality, life and vigour. Be careful to choose a green of the right intensity for you. Yellow is a sunshine colour, full of warmth and light. Red is a very sexual colour, difficult to live with for most people, and you must get the lighting right otherwise it can be garish.

Pink, as mentioned earlier, is a gentle colour of romance and love and is a comforting hue. Purple and lilac are associated with power and inspiration.

Smell is also very important, so be generous with a spray of your favourite perfume on the sheet — but not too generous, as any perfume can become stifling in excess. Flowers are always wonderful in a bedroom, especially those which give off a gentle scent. Daffodils, winter aconites, lilies, old-fashioned roses or freesias, are all charming in the bedroom. And there is something agreeably decadent about having flowers near where you sleep — they can make you feel quite pampered.

Don't rely on a single ceiling light to illuminate your room, as it will cast a gloomy functional glow over everything. Small bedside lamps mean you don't have to get cold toes. A thick white church candle on a solid base is perfect for relaxing you, and when making love by the gentle glow of candlelight, you will look at your best.

Ideally, your should do very little in the half hour before you sleep so that you can wind down. That also means not reading anything that will stimulate your brain into thinking about something new. If you do want to play music, choose something gentle and soothing, perhaps some New Age or classical music which gives the impression of being never-ending.

Avoid clutter in your bedroom, keep it clean and air it every day by opening the window. Do not take work into your bedroom. Keep it just for dreaming, sleeping and making love.

Your bedroom will become a haven of peace and your understanding of the dreams you have there will enhance your life.

NOTES

NOTES

NOTES

NOTES

NOTES

NOTES